ACKNOWLEDGMENTS

A book of this scope cannot be created without the help of many people. To make sure we had the latest information, we leaned heavily on various government agencies as well as private organizations. But institutions don't respond to pleas for help; it's the individuals within these organizations who follow through. The authors gratefully acknowledge the cooperation and assistance of the following organizations and the people who make them work:

AGENCY FOR TOXIC SUBSTANCES AND DISEASE REGISTRY
Lydia Ogden Askew and Barry L. Johnson

CENTERS FOR DISEASE CONTROL
Mary M. Agocs, Sue Binder, Robert C. Diefenbach, Christie Ehema, Ruth A. Etzel, Anita Highsmith, Dennis Juranek, Mark McClanahan, and William Roper, CDC Administrator

CONSUMER PRODUCT SAFETY COMMISSION
Ken Chiles, Sandra Eberle, Mary Marshal, Bill Mensa, and Susan Womble

ENVIRONMENTAL PROTECTION AGENCY
Bob Axelrad, Betsy Agle, Michael A. Berry, Jackie Bishop, Jerome Blondell, Gwen Brown, Martha Casey, Lew Crampton, Frank Davido, Susan Dillman, James Elder, Elissa Feldman, Carl Grable, Clare Grubbs, Richard Guimond, Karen Hoffman, Kelly

Leovic, David Mundari, Michelle Price, Jeanne Richards, Janet Remmers, Joe Schechter, Tom Tillman, Jim Quackenboss, and Lance A. Wallace

U.S. DEPARTMENT OF ENERGY
Jon Talbott, David Moses, and Susan Rose

U.S. DEPARTMENT OF HOUSING AND URBAN DEVELOPMENT (HUD)
Dick Alexander and Ellis Goldman

STATE GOVERNMENT OFFICIALS
Alabama—Jim McVay
Arizona—Shane Siren
Arkansas—Stanley Evans
California—James A. Arteaga, Department of Health Services; Peggy Vanicek, Product Division of the California Air Resources Board; Greg Thompson, Attorney General's Office
Delaware—Sheri L. Woodruff
Florida—Anita Durham
Iowa—Jack Kelly
Indiana—Mary Ann McKinney
Kentucky—Brad Hughes
Louisiana—Gwen Bach-Stewart
Michigan—Ute von der Heyden
Mississippi—Nancy Kay Sullivan
Montana—Charles Aagenes
Nevada—Donald Kwalick, M.D., M.P.H.
New Mexico—William M. Floyd, M.S.
New York—Peter Slocum
North Carolina—Don Follmer
South Dakota—Barbara E. Buhler
Tennessee—Suellen Joyner
Vermont—Linda Fox Dorey
West Virginia—Ann Garcelon
Wisconsin—Jay Goldring and Linda Knobeloch
Wyoming—Helen G. Levine

NONGOVERNMENTAL EXPERTS
J. R. Beckman, Ph.D., Arizona State University, Tempe, AZ; Sharon Blair, media coordinator at the Bonneville Power Admin-

istration; Geary Campbell, International Bottled Water Association; Gary Havens, Editor, *Family Handyman* magazine; David E. Jacobs, an environmental research scientist and John Toon, communications officer, at Georgia Tech Research Institute and Georgia Institute of Technology; Anthony Giometti, American Society of Heating, Refrigerating, and Air Conditioning Engineers; Dr. Arthur M. Langer, Environmental Sciences Laboratory, City University of New York; Dr. Melvin Reuber, National Coalition Against the Misuse of Pesticides.

ALSO IMPORTANT

American Academy of Otolaryngic Allergy, American College of Allergy and Immunology, American Medical Association, Asthma and Allergy Foundation of America, Doctor's Data, Foundation for Allergy Care and Treatment, National Center for Health Statistics, National Institute of Allergy and Infectious Diseases, National Jewish Center for Immunology and Respiratory Medicine, U.S. Department of Agriculture.

The Breecher Alabama support crew: My (MMB) wife, Rebecca Oxford, Ph.D., for her encouragement and patience; her graduate students—Kathleen Barnard, Diana Horton-Murillo and Kim Young—for library research and proofreading skills. Also Michelle Clements, Bob Johnson, and David Benson for clerical and production support.

Last, but certainly not least, the John Wiley & Sons, Inc. editorial staff, our editor Steve Ross, and his assistant, Alexandra White, as well as the scores of other individuals involved in manufacturing, promoting, and otherwise marketing this book.

Maury M. Breecher, M.P.H.
Tuscaloosa, Alabama

Shirley Linde, Ph.D.
Tierra Verde, Florida

CONTENTS

CHAPTER 1

WARNING

Your Home May Be Hazardous to Your Health

Home seems to be such a safe place. We picture it as a haven, a place to which we can escape from the dangers of the world, much as our ancestors escaped the saber-toothed tiger by clustering around their campfires. We can easily picture the ideal home where the family gathers around the warmth of the fireplace, windows and doors tightly closed against a wintry storm, father with his pipe, mother with her sewing, a dog at their feet. But something is fundamentally wrong with this picture.

Our homes may now be terribly hazardous to our health. We may be drinking troubled waters, breathing air inside the house that is more dangerous than the air downwind of an industrial city, or absorbing chemicals that cause fatigue, listlessness, headaches, and other symptoms. We may also be exposed to hidden radiation over long periods that could cause death. And the situation is occurring not just in a few houses near hazardous waste dumps, but in old houses, new houses, country cottages, suburban houses, city apartments, and million-dollar mansions across the nation. Almost no home is immune, whether it's 100 years old or recently built.

The possibility was even considered in the White House. In 1991 doctors ordered an analysis of water supplies at the White House and other presidential and vice-presidential residences to see if they contained chemicals that could have triggered the thyroid disease afflicting both President and Mrs. Bush and the autoimmune disease of their dog Millie. Some elevated lead levels *were* found. It highlighted in many people's minds for the first time that hidden poisons

1

can indeed be present even in the most expensive and prestigious homes, even in what is probably the most-looked-after house in the nation.

The Culprits

How widespread is the problem of our houses being able to make us sick? What health problems can be caused? Here are some of the frightening truths.

RADON GAS   Millions of families are being exposed to dangerous—sometimes deadly—levels of radon gas. In fact, studies by the Environmental Protection Agency (EPA) indicate that as many as 10 percent of all American homes may have elevated levels of radon, and the percentage may be higher in some geographic areas. Radon is now known to be the nation's second leading cause of lung cancer. Indeed, the EPA estimates that some 16,000 Americans die every year from lung cancer caused by radon. According to an article in *Science* magazine, the health risks from breathing radon are even higher than from smoking cigarettes. And if a person exposed to radon is also a smoker, the risk of lung cancer is increased by at least tenfold! This report was released by the prestigious National Research Council after a comprehensive, three-year study funded by the EPA and the Nuclear Regulatory Commission.

> The federal government recommends that you measure the level of radon in your house or apartment. The agencies listed in Directory A at the back of this book can provide information and instruction.

LEAD   In addition, many of us may unknowingly be exposing ourselves to dangerous amounts of lead. The effects of lead poisoning have been known for years, but only recently have we learned how widespread lead contamination is. It isn't just the old house with peeling paint that holds danger of lead poisoning. Houses of all types—perhaps one in five, in all areas—can have lead contamination. Symptoms come not only from eating paint chips, but also from inhaling lead dust in the air. The symptoms, found at all ages, include such diverse effects as learning disabilities and behavioral problems in children; arthritis-like joint pains, stomach pains, or high blood pressure in adults; and irritability, fatigue, and damage to brain, kidney, and nervous systems in anyone. Many studies have shown that children with elevated lead levels have lower IQ scores, have poorer scores on auditory and language functioning, and often have difficulties paying attention. The most recent studies show that lower mental development in children caused by lead poisoning is so common that a number of groups now recommend that all children aged one or two be tested for lead in their bodies as part of their early pediatric checkups. Think about the effect this could be having: A drop in a child's intelligence and ability not only affects that individual family, but when there are large numbers of children exposed to lead, as there are today, the broader implications for society are staggering.

Could you be exposed to lead and not know it? Indeed, millions of people, especially pregnant women and children, are at risk. Lead in house paints was banned years ago, but many houses still have old paint. Water may contain lead because of lead pipes in old houses or because lead is sometimes still used when soldering plumbing joints in new homes. You can also inhale lead from automobile exhaust fumes in your garage or from a nearby highway.

"The news on lead is getting worse—lead is the nation's no. 1 environmental threat to the health of children."

Louis Sullivan M.D., Secretary of the U.S. Department of Health and Human Services.

FORMALDEHYDE Formaldehyde may be another danger lurking in your house. High concentrations of formaldehyde have been shown to cause cancer in animals and probably also cause cancer in humans. Low levels can result in breathing problems, dizziness, eye and skin irritations, nausea, headaches, and heart palpitations. Formaldehyde is found in most homes since it's given off by particle-board building material and some furniture, carpet backing and other flooring, and permanent-press clothing.

ASBESTOS Do you have asbestos in your home? Asbestos, found in dozens of home building materials, is a well-publicized cause of cancer in humans. Until the mid-70s asbestos was widely used as an insulation and building material because of its fire resistance. However, medical evidence that was first reported in 1972 showed that asbestos could cause cancer and degenerative lung disease (similar to emphysema). Epidemiologists at Harvard University School of Public Health estimate that within the next 20 years some 70,000 more people will get cancer and that almost an equal number will get serious lung disease because of their exposure to asbestos. At last count, more that 30,000 people had sued one asbestos company because they became ill from breathing in asbestos fibers. Thousands of other suits have been filed against other companies. Some are settled; some are still pending.

WATER CONTAMINANTS   We can no longer assume that even our drinking water is safe. For too long people have taken for granted that the water they are drinking from their taps is pure and fresh. The truth is it may be making us sick. From Florida to California, municipal wells have been found to be contaminated by industrial solvents, fuel from leaking tanks, agricultural pesticides, and toxic chemicals. In many places there are unacceptable levels of benzene, lead, and cadmium in the drinking water. Even good-tasting water can be toxic.

In one New England town, residents were told not to drink their water because it was contaminated with asbestos. On a farm in Washington State a man died of cancer, children were sick, family dogs and cats died. When the Environmental Protection Agency tested the well water, they found that it was being contaminated with chemicals from cleaning solvents at a nearby waste dump. In Massachusetts, an estimated 8,000 people became ill with diarrhea when the parasite *Giardia* made its way into the town water supply. In a southern coastal town, residents were without water for more than a month because of greenish-brown slime coming from the taps. A lubricating oil had contaminated their system. Sales are booming for bottled water and filters.

AIR POLLUTION   The air in your house or apartment may also be making you sick. Indoor pollution is believed responsible for the huge increase in hospitalizations for asthma—an increase of 50 percent for adults and 200 percent for children in the past 20 years. Gas fumes can lead to headaches, nausea, and fatigue; carbon monoxide and other fumes can leak into homes from cars and chemicals in attached garages. The levels of nitrogen dioxide and carbon monoxide in homes often exceed the *outdoor* limits set by the federal government.

"Your home may be more of a toxic waste hazard than Love Canal or the chemical company nearby."

Lance Wallace, Ph.D., Office of Research and Development, Environmental Protection Agency, Warrenton VA.

A Major Worldwide Health Problem

Air pollutants, pesticides, fuels, solvents, fumes, heavy metals, radon, asbestos—the list of toxic substances found in most of our homes is long. Formerly sprayed in homes for termites, the pesticide chlordane, which has been proved to cause cancer in animals, persists for 20 years or more; it was used in 30 million homes.

We breathe fumes from detergents and disinfectants under the kitchen sink, hair sprays, underarm deodorants, colognes, air fresheners, nail polish, floor waxes and polishes, moth flakes, insect sprays, paints, turpentines, varnishes. If your garage is attached to the house, you may have the added problem of car exhaust fumes adding to the pollution. Just starting the car and backing it out will produce fumes that can seep up into the house for the rest of the day; in addition there are fumes from the carburetor, the gasoline tank, oil leaks, and from lawn mower gasoline and oil. A trip to the dry cleaners or the gas station can leave you with the residue of tetrachloroethylene or benzene on your breath for hours. The damage all these fumes cause is just beginning to come to light. The effects may be devastatingly serious.

"Polychlorinated biphenyls (PCBs), dioxin, and asbestos are now among the toxic materials whose common use in earlier years has left a legacy of contamination that plagues wide areas of the country today . . . PCBs were widely used for about 50 years because of their heat resistant properties. So persistent is this group of chemicals that everyone in this country likely has trace levels of it in their bodies."

Environmental Protection Agency.

A committee of The World Health Organization estimates that as many as one in three new or remodeled buildings may have "sick building" problems. Experts estimate that from 5 to 15 million people in the United States alone may be affected. The truth is that we really don't know, because the number of sufferers increases constantly as new chemicals are introduced into the home. The American Academy of Environmental Medicine estimates that some 60,000 new chemical combinations are manufactured *every month!*

Many people have developed supersensitivities in which their bodies seem to react to even small exposures of common chemicals such as household cleaners, perfumes, and food additives. Often the condition goes unrecognized, but the person just feels lifeless and tired, has headaches, stomachaches, or more infections than other people.

All of our homes—including yours—have the potential to make us sick. Sometimes it's just a little bit of exposure, but that little bit of exposure every day can make you sick. And the worst part of the nightmare is that the hazards often are hidden and silent. You can't smell or see or taste them, but every time you walk through your front door you may be bombarded by them. Since most of us spend 90 to 95 percent of our time indoors (21 to 23 hours a day indoors), the hidden hazards relentlessly work on our bodies and may ultimately wreck our health.

The truth is that there are people all over the country thinking "I can't shake this cold" when it's their house that is making them sick. And many times the symptoms are more serious—behavior problems, kidney damage, relentless fatigue.

And even beyond that, many experts say that at low doses, even far below the level at which one can detect obvious symptoms, toxic substances can be causing harm.

A joint guide published by the EPA and the U.S. Consumer Product Safety Commission, says that health effects from indoor air pollutants fall into two categories: those that are experienced immediately after exposure and those that do not show up until years later.

"Immediate effects, which may show up after a single exposure or repeated exposures, include irritation of the eyes, nose, and throat, headaches, dizziness, and fatigue. These immediate effects are usually short-term and treatable by some means. Sometimes the treatment is simply eliminating the person's exposure to the source of the pollution, if it can be identified. Other health effects may show up either years after exposure has occurred or only after long or repeated periods of exposure."

The Consumer Federation of America calls our sick houses the "number 1 health and safety issue of our time," adding billions to the nation's health bill.

The Sick Building Syndrome Moves Home

How did it happen that housing evolved to the point where your home could hurt you?

Part of the problem is due to the increasing number of chemicals used in building and maintaining our homes, but part of the problem is also that, in the past, most buildings had air flow from open windows, air leaks, and building materials that breathed. Now with air-conditioning and with tight construction and extra insulation to conserve energy in the energy crisis, and with many people leaving their houses closed all day and night, the pollutants in the house build up, often to health-threatening levels. We first began to hear of "sick building syndrome" in the early 1980s when architects and builders began to create airtight insulated office buildings to keep heat in and cold out. As the tightness trapped hazardous fumes in poorly ventilated spaces, workers developed headaches, burning eyes, and breathing problems from their sealed environments. Now those same problems are spreading to homes.

Tight weather-stripping and caulking make for energy-efficient houses, but with formaldehyde, cigarette smoke, oven fumes, and other pollutants, energy-*efficient* can become health-*deficient*.

As outside air is kept out, household pollutants are sealed in, and recent research indicates they are having more significant effects than ever before suspected.

As we spend more and more time at home (now we even have a name for it — cocooning), we are increasingly at risk to the hazards. Remember Legionnaires' disease? It was one of the first examples of building-related sickness and was caused by a bacteria growing in an air-conditioning system. Now, according to an article in the *Journal of the American Medical Association*, researchers have found that as many as 30 percent of homes in some communities may have water systems contaminated with the same germ.

A Sick House Can Be Cured

The good news is that there are things you can do to make your home safe again. You can find the hidden hazards in your home and take steps to counteract them. This book will show you how. We urge you to follow its program. Your health and your family's health are at stake.

> "A sensible guide would surely be to reduce exposure to hazard whenever possible, to accept substantial hazard only for great benefit, minor hazard for modest benefit, and no hazard at all when the benefit seems relatively trivial."
>
> *Dr. Philip Handler, late former director, the National Academy of Sciences.*

You can make your home healthier and safer, if you know what to look for and what to do about any problems that you find. We will bring you the knowledge that you need from leading authorities of groups such as the Environmental Protection Agency, the Centers for Disease Control, the Agency for Toxic Substances and Disease Registry, and the Consumer Product Safety Commission.

We will tell you when to take asbestos out and when it's less dangerous to leave it in, how to test for radon seeping from the ground, and how to find the hidden formaldehyde, toxic wastes, and other dangers in your home that you clean with, paint with, eat and sleep with.

And we will give you step-by-step directions and guidelines for correcting the problems. We'll tell you about products to test your home and to clean up your air and water, what to do about radon, asbestos, formaldehyde, and lead. We'll tell you how and where to dispose of hazardous wastes. And we'll give you lists of associations, governmental agencies, and foundations that supply further information and local help.

In fact, we will bring together all the pertinent information concerning sick house syndrome, giving advice from the most authoritative experts in the nation, pointing out controversies where controversies exist, and giving details of the latest studies. All this information will help you determine whether your house could be making *you* sick, causing your tiredness, your child's constant runny nose, your spouse's headaches, and all the other symptoms of sick house syndrome, from which millions of people are suffering.

The important thing is that a sick house can be cured. You can exert control over your personal environment and make the simple changes that can ensure your, and your family's, future safety and well-being. We want you to have a healing house or apartment, a place where you can come safely to renew yourself.

It's time to call for a home ecology revolution, to take control of our home environments and to change them to the safe, healthy havens they should be. Just as people are thinking of the outside environment and about the food they put in their bodies, we need to start thinking about our homes and the health of our home environment. It's time to bring the environmental movement indoors.

The Safe-at-Home Health Inventory

Step one when starting to make your house safe is to take a health inventory of yourself and the members of your family.

Think over any symptoms that you or your family have been having. Go over the following list and check off any symptoms that are persistent or seem to recur frequently.

- ☐ Headaches
- ☐ Stomachache or nausea
- ☐ Sneezing
- ☐ Itchy, red, or irritated eyes
- ☐ Skin rashes
- ☐ Fatigue
- ☐ Dizziness
- ☐ Drowsiness
- ☐ Breathing problems
- ☐ Persistent coughs
- ☐ Insomnia
- ☐ Joint pains
- ☐ Dry or irritated throat
- ☐ Sinus congestion
- ☐ Confusion
- ☐ Irritability
- ☐ Inability to concentrate
- ☐ Behavior problems
- ☐ Just feeling bad but aren't sick enough to go to bed

They can all be due to unhealthy conditions in your house. You should be especially suspicious of the symptoms being caused by your home if your symptoms started when you moved into a new house or when you recently remodeled or refurnished, or if you find that your symptoms get better or disappear when you leave your home, particularly when you go away for several days.

If you're one of the people frequently suffering some of these symptoms, the chances are excellent that the Safe-at-Home program will help make those symptoms disappear or at least become less intense.

You can create a safe home environment. Instead of living in a house that could make you sick, we want you to have a healing house, one that is free of pollution and hazards where you and your family can live in health.

CHAPTER 2

RADON GAS

A Deadly Threat to Millions

In autumn of 1984, Stan Watras discovered that his family's home in Boyertown, Pennsylvania, had been visited by a silent and deadly intruder—radon.

Watras worked at a nuclear power plant, and one day, about a year after moving into his new home, he mysteriously started setting off radiation detectors when he went to work. Authorities scrambled to trace the source of his "body radiation" and were eventually stunned to discover it was his home.

Radiation specialists measured radon levels in the Watras home and discovered the highest residential radon level ever found up to that time—2,700 pCi/L—almost 2,000 times higher than the "average" levels found in most homes! Stan and his family had been living in the middle of a radioactive cloud. Experts told him and his family that the amount of radiation they had received over a one-year period was equal to 545,000 chest x-rays, that they had a 585 percent greater chance of developing lung cancer than other families, and that the potential damage to their lungs was equal to smoking 220 packs of cigarettes a day.

Radon is a naturally occurring radioactive gas that seeps from bedrock and ground into homes and buildings. It can enter your home through cracks in the foundation, floor drains, sumps, joints, and tiny cracks or pores in hollow-block concrete walls. The threat posed by radon is unseen and unfelt, and the risk occurs in that most unlikely and trusted of places—our homes.

Millions of Homes Are at Risk from Radon
Eight to ten million American dwellings have unhealthy basement radiation levels greater than 4 pCi/L (picocuries per liter of air), according to the Environmental Protection Agency (EPA).

Radon Can Be Deadly

The air inside the average U.S. home contains radon amounting to about 1.5 picocuries per liter, but "averages" are misleading. If 1.5 pCi/L is "average," that means that 50 percent of us have "above average" levels and therefore an above average risk of having adverse health effects due to radon. Even the slightly higher level of 2 pCi/L is equal to about 200 chest x-rays per year. Roughly one out of 100 people exposed to 2 pCi/L over a lifetime will develop lung cancer. If you apply this average to a very conservative estimate of 10 million people exposed to 2 pCi/L over a lifetime, that is 100,000 cases of lung cancer.

So, if that is the case, then what does the 4 pCi/L level mean? The EPA has established that level as a rough guideline—a point above which it recommends that the public take specific follow-up actions. The agency is *not* telling people that levels of 4 pCi/L and lower are "safe" or might not still lead to increased incidences of lung cancer. Rather, the EPA says the 4 pCi/L figure is a guide for people to use in deciding *how much* risk they care to accept.

The risk of lung cancer from radon exposure depends on two factors: the *level* of radon to which one is exposed and the *duration of exposure* to the silent killer. Even with relatively low levels, if you are exposed to radon for a long time it can be deadly.

The 4 pCi/L level "still has a fair amount of risk," said Richard Guimond, former director of EPA's Office of Radiation. He warned that the level of 4 pCi/L is almost the same as smoking one-half pack of cigarettes a day. To put the 4 pCi/L level further into perspective, it's helpful to know that the risk represented by that level compares to having 400 chest x-rays per year! Roughly two out of 100 people exposed to that level over a lifetime would get lung cancer. The risks to smokers are even greater because of the interaction (synergistic effect) of the two cancer causers.

If your home has radon levels that test between 2 pCi/L and 4 pCi/L, you may want to consider taking action to reduce those levels even further. The EPA strongly urges people with readings higher than 4 pCi/L to confirm the readings with further tests and, if duplicated, to take action to reduce radon below that level. Necessary action usually involves routine construction or repair work.

"This is a serious problem," says Margo T. Oge, director of the EPA's radon division. "Radon is invisible. People can't see, taste, or smell it. Rather, it lurks silently in the background, working its mischief only after years of exposure."

Dr. Charles Dudney, of the Oak Ridge National Laboratory in Tennessee, calls radon the most serious cancer-causing agent in the environment.

Radon's "mischief" is deadly. The National Academy of Sciences estimates that radon-caused lung cancer already costs the United States some 16,000 deaths annually. Therefore it is extremely important to determine the levels of radon in your own home. We'll tell you more about home testing in a moment. First, we'll give some background on what radon is and where it comes from.

Radon Is One of the Worst Health Risks We Face

"Radon is one of the larger health risks people face," says Richard Guimond, former director of the EPA's Office of Radiation. "It is the second most prevalent cause of lung cancer. Youngsters and anyone who smokes are particularly at risk."

Radon and Where It Comes From

Radon is an invisible, odorless, radioactive gas produced by the decay of uranium in rock and soil. This radioactive gas leaks through bedrock and percolates up through the ground. It can be found at various concentrations practically anywhere on earth, but when concentrations accumulate in closed buildings, health risks become a concern. Once airborne, the radioactive particles attach themselves to dust. This deadly dust, if inhaled, can cause damage to lung tissue and increase one's chances of lung cancer.

Radon readings tend to be highest in areas with high concentrations of uranium-bearing rocks. Rock usually contains about 2.7 pounds of uranium for every million pounds. However, some kinds of rock contain more uranium than others. Granite, for instance, has

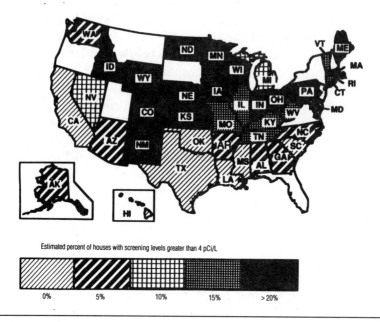

Estimated percent of houses with screening levels greater than 4 pCi/L

0%   5%   10%   15%   > 20%

State/EPA radon survey. These results represent two-to-seven-day *screening* measurements and should not be used to estimate annual averages or health risks.

about 4.7 pounds uranium per million pounds. For that reason, the "Reading Prong," a geographic area extending through the granite-rich mid-Atlantic states of Pennsylvania and New Jersey, has perilously high radon levels.

The EPA also found high levels in Minnesota and North Dakota, where 46 and 63 percent, respectively, of the homes screened were found to have levels above the 4 pCi/L guideline. Check the map, *State/EPA radon survey.* But don't be lulled into a false sense of security if your state appears to be in a low-radon area. Scientists caution that although there are geological "hot spots," radon problems have been found in every state in the union.

How to Test for Radon in Your Home

Radon strikes capriciously; it can creep into and accumulate high levels in one home while the house next door remains unscathed. That's why it is important for *everyone* to test for radon.

Since there are over 300 different firms manufacturing and selling radon test kits, you as a consumer have to be careful in choosing one. Although the United States does not have a national program to certify radon measurement companies, the EPA Office of Radiation's Radon Division does have a program to determine the accuracy of radon detectors. Companies submit their radon detection devices for evaluation on a voluntary basis to the EPA's Radon Measurement Proficiency (RMP) program. Companies that have passed the RMP evaluation will generally publicize that fact on their device or in the literature accompanying it. If not, consumers can contact the radon office of their state's health department or one of the EPA's regional offices to double-check whether the radon detection device they want to purchase has passed the EPA's proficiency evaluation. (See Directory A at the back of this book to find the phone number of a radon office in your state or see Directory B for the number of one of the EPA's regional offices). *Consumer Reports* magazine has published two excellent articles on radon, one in July 1987 and the other in October 1989. For reprints of the articles, write Consumers Union, 101 Truman Ave, Yonkers NY 10703. They also published a noteworthy book, *Radon: A Homeowner's Guide to Detection and Control,* in 1987.

To determine whether your family is at risk, you should first do a screening measurement using a radon detection device that has passed muster with the EPA's RMP program. Devices usually cost from $10 to $50 and are available at hardware stores or can be ordered by phone directly from the various manufacturing companies. We recommend that you order your radon testing kit by phone because you can't tell how long the kit may have stayed on a store's shelf.

The two most popular types of commercially available radon detectors are the charcoal canister (either a charcoal adsorption detector or diffusion barrier charcoal adsorption detector) and the alpha track detector. Both charcoal and alpha track detectors work by being exposed to the air in your home for a specified period of time, usually 48 hours. After the time has passed, you send the detection device to a specified laboratory for analysis. The cost of the analysis is included in the cost of the kit.

Although the alpha track detector is a popular detector, it did not perform well in a University of Iowa study that compared 15 different types of detectors. According to the study, published in the *American Journal of Public Health,* charcoal adsorption detectors and diffusion barrier charcoal adsorption detectors performed best. The two top-performing radon detectors contained "diffusion barriers," which keep out moisture and radioactive materials other than radon. This is important but rarely reported information.

STEP ONE—THE SCREENING MEASUREMENT   The initial screening measurement should be made in the lived-in area of your home that is closest to the ground. (There is no need to check basements unless you have basement bedrooms, recreation rooms, or workshops and spend a great deal of time there.) For at least 12 hours prior to the start of the test, all windows and doors should be closed and should be kept closed throughout the 48-hour testing period to keep the radon level relatively constant throughout the testing period. Because of the need to keep the windows closed as much as possible, the EPA recommends that you make short-term radon measurements during cool months of the year, because in the summer the use of an air conditioner or open windows could lower the readings. Once you send the radon detection devices to the laboratory, you should get the results back within one or two weeks.

To interpret the results, you must understand that radon, a gaseous decay product of uranium, decays further, emitting solid isotopes of polonium. These polonium isotopes emit high-energy, low-velocity particles called alpha radiation. Alpha particles constantly bombard our bodies yet cause no harm, as most cannot penetrate our skin. But breathed deep into the lungs, these polonium isotopes radiate alpha particles directly into sensitive and vulnerable lung tissue. The effects may not be seen for years or even decades, but the damage can cause lung cancer. Results from the tests will be reported in one of two ways. Results from test kits that measure concentrations of radon report in units known as picocuries per liter—the pCi/L measurement. One picocurie per liter represents the decay of about two radon atoms per minute in one liter of air. Results from test kits that measure radon decay products are reported in arbitrary units of measurement known as "working levels" (WL). One working level of radon decay products roughly corresponds to the amount of radon decay products released by 200 pCi/L of radon in the air.

The *Radon risk evaluation chart* shows a wide range of exposure levels and the associated risk of death from lung cancer.

STEP TWO—INTERPRETING THE SCREENING MEASUREMENT AND DETERMINING THE NEED FOR FOLLOW-UP TESTS   The step one screening method described is a short-term method that gives you a quick

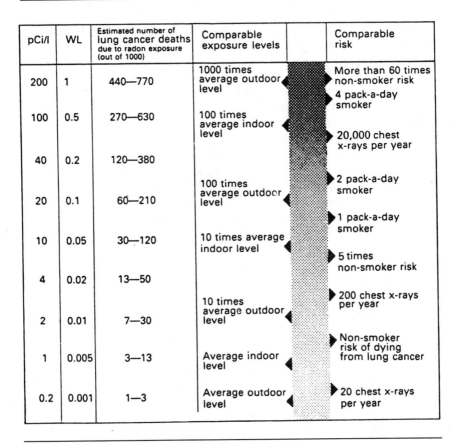

pCi/l	WL	Estimated number of lung cancer deaths due to radon exposure (out of 1000)	Comparable exposure levels		Comparable risk
200	1	440—770	1000 times average outdoor level		More than 60 times non-smoker risk
					4 pack-a-day smoker
100	0.5	270—630	100 times average indoor level		
					20,000 chest x-rays per year
40	0.2	120—380			
			100 times average outdoor level		2 pack-a-day smoker
20	0.1	60—210			
					1 pack-a-day smoker
10	0.05	30—120	10 times average indoor level		
					5 times non-smoker risk
4	0.02	13—50			
			10 times average outdoor level		200 chest x-rays per year
2	0.01	7—30			
					Non-smoker risk of dying from lung cancer
1	0.005	3—13	Average indoor level		
0.2	0.001	1—3	Average outdoor level		20 chest x-rays per year

Radon risk evaluation chart. To clearly understand the relative seriousness of exposure to radon, this chart shows how exposure to various levels over a lifetime compares to the risk of developing fatal lung cancer from smoking and from chest x-rays. The chart also compares these levels to the average indoor and outdoor radon concentrations. (*Source: A Citizen's Guide to Radon*, U.S. Government Printing Office, 1989.)

and inexpensive idea of whether or not you have a potential radon problem. However, it's not the most reliable measure of the *long-term* radon exposure to which you and your family may be exposed. Since radon levels can vary greatly from season to season as well as from room to room, the step one screening measurement only serves to indicate the *potential* for a radon problem. Depending on the results of your screening measurement, you may need to have follow-up measurements made.

The EPA offers the following advice as an aid to determining the urgency of your need for follow-up measurements:

> If your screening measurement result is greater than about 1.0 WL or greater than about 200 pCi/L, you should perform follow-up measurements as soon as possible. Expose the follow-up detectors for no more than one week. Doors and windows should be closed as much as possible during testing. You should also consider taking action to immediately reduce the radon levels in your home.
>
> If your screening measurement result is about 0.1 WL to about 1.0 WL or about 20 pCi/L to about 200 pCi/L, perform follow-up measurements by exposing detectors for no more than three months. Again, doors and windows should be closed as much as possible during testing.
>
> If your screening measurement result is about 0.02 WL to about 0.1 WL or about 4 pCi/L, follow-up measurements are probably not required. If the screening measurement was made with the house closed up prior to and during the testing period, there is relatively little chance that the radon concentration in your home will be greater than 0.02 WL or 4 pCi/L as an annual average.

How to interpret results of follow-up tests. The results of your follow-up measurements provide you with an idea of the average radon gas concentration throughout your home. The actual risk you face depends on the amount of time you are exposed to this concentration. The illustration *Indoor radon risk* gives a representation of the numbers of lung cancer deaths out of a group of 100 people that scientists would attribute to exposure to specific levels of indoor radon. The estimates assume that these 100 persons spent 75 percent of their time in the dwelling for 70 years. Each of the four estimates of mortality is *in addition to* the numbers of lung cancer deaths attributed to other causes.

Although the risks posed by high radon concentrations constitute "bad news," the "good news" lies in the fact that those risks can be reduced—without huge outlays of money or extensive lifestyle changes. In a way, the Watras family was lucky to have found out about their exposure so early. They experienced ultra-high levels of radon for only a year and were able to take action to reduce the levels of radon in their home, thus lowering their long-term risk. In fact, their home was used as a "test home" by the federal government to see if ultra-high radon levels could be reduced. They were reduced to a daily average of 4 pCi/L. The Watras family still lives in the same home.

Risk of lung cancer death caused by radon in people living for 70 years in houses having various levels of radon:

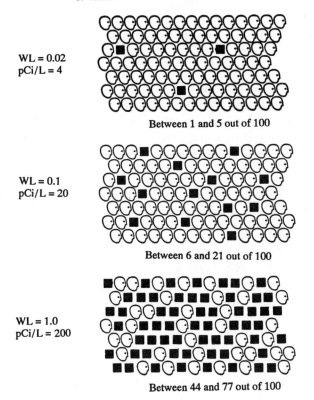

WL = 0.02
pCi/L = 4

Between 1 and 5 out of 100

WL = 0.1
pCi/L = 20

Between 6 and 21 out of 100

WL = 1.0
pCi/L = 200

Between 44 and 77 out of 100

If these same 100 individuals had lived only 10 years (instead of 70) in houses with radon levels of about 1.0 WL, the number of lung cancer deaths expected would be:

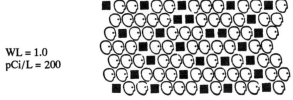

WL = 1.0
pCi/L = 200

Between 14 and 42 out of 100

Indoor radon risk. (*Source: A Citizen's Guide to Radon,* U.S. Government Printing Office, 1989.)

When to Take Action

You too can lower your long-term risk from radon. If follow-up measurements confirm elevated radon levels in the living areas of your house, the EPA recommends the following take-action time frames:

- Less than 4 pCi/L or 0.02 WL: Although radon levels in this range may represent a significant health risk, cost-effective reduction methods to get below this range are limited. However, increasing ventilation and limiting the time spent in areas of the house with higher radon concentrations may help reduce the risks.
- 4 to 20 pCi/L or 0.02 to 0.1 WL: Action should be taken to reduce radon levels as low as possible within a year or two.
- 20 to 200 pCi/L or 0.1 to 1.0 WL: Exposures at this range are among the highest ever measured. Action should be undertaken to reduce radon levels as far as possible within several weeks. If this is not feasible, a temporary increase in ventilation or temporary relocation should be considered.

The cure for this

Simple Solutions

Although each home poses unique radon reduction challenges, everyone can reduce his or her risk from radon by taking the following four simple steps.

1. Spend less time in areas of high concentrations of radon, generally low areas, such as the basement.
2. Whenever practical, open all windows and turn on fans to increase the air flow into and through the house. This is especially important in the basement.
3. If your home has a crawl space beneath it, keep the crawl-space vents on all sides of the house fully open all year.
4. Stop smoking and discourage smoking by others in your home. By stopping smoking, you not only reduce your family's overall chance of developing lung cancer, you also eliminate the synergistic (multiplied) effect of the carcinogenic compounds in smoke and the cancer-causing potential of radon.

Four Permanent and Cost-Effective Radon Solutions

Remember, your risk of lung cancer from exposure to radon depends on two factors: the amount of radon entering your home and the length of time you are exposed. There are four major ways to permanently reduce radon in your home. They are identified based on their operating principles:

1. Suctioning radon gas from the soil (using any of three distinct suction methods: subslab, drain tile, and block wall)
2. Sealing off radon entry routes
3. Controlling air pressure in the house
4. Increasing house ventilation

The first three are preventive methods, and the last is an after-the-fact response to radon. The methods are often used in combination for greater results. The cost, complexity, and potential for reducing radon levels vary considerably among the four methods. Selecting the right radon reduction method for your own house can be a complicated decision. Before making that decision, let's explore the three methods of preventing radon entry. We'll discuss the fourth method, increasing ventilation to reduce radon, in Chapter 4.

SUCTIONING RADON FROM THE SOIL   The most widely used of all radon reduction methods is soil gas suction because it effectively prevents radon from entering the home. Soil gas suction works by drawing radon away from under and around the house, before it can enter.

Soil gas suction techniques are most successful for houses with what technicians refer to as "good subslab permeability." Material with a large particle size, such as clean, coarse gravel, is more permeable than a material of small particle size, such as clay soil. In other words, suction works best if you have gravel under your foundation.

The objective of soil gas suction is to reduce the air pressure under the house's concrete slab (or on its block walls) to a pressure lower than that inside the house. This lower air pressure reverses the flow of radon. Instead of seeping into the house, it is sucked out. The following paragraphs will describe the three types of soil gas suction.

Subslab suction. This method involves installing pipes and fans. The fans are connected to the pipes (ducts) so as to draw the soil gas out from under the house. Fans are commonly located in an attic area or the exterior of the house. Subslab suction is generally considered the most effective radon reduction technique because it can reduce radon levels by 80 to 99 percent when permeability underneath the slab is good.

Subslab suction systems can be installed by professionals for about $1,000 to $2,000. The exhaust fans use electricity that adds an operating cost of about $140 per year.

Although *not* a simple do-it-yourself job, homeowners with the necessary skills and equipment have successfully installed subslab suction systems, saving hundreds of dollars in labor costs. Materials including fans and polyvinylchloride (PVC) pipes will cost $300 to $400. If you want to consider the do-it-yourself approach, write the EPA for their technical manual *Radon Reduction Techniques for Detached Houses: Technical Guidance.* The manual provides detailed information on the selection, design, and installation of radon reduction systems. This manual is primarily for the professional radon reduction contractor or the very skilled do-it-yourself homeowner. For homes with crawl spaces, refer to the drawing *Two suction techniques for under the house.*

An advantage of subslab suction is that the installation of pipes and fans can be combined with either or both of the next two methods.

Drain tile suction. At some houses, water is directed away from the foundation by perforated pipes (drain tiles) installed alongside the foundation of the house. The tiles usually drain either to an above-grade discharge spot located away from the house, or to an internal sump. If these drain tiles form a complete loop around the exterior or interior of the home's footing, they may be used to draw radon away from the surrounding soil and reduce or prevent radon entry into the house.

If the tiles drain to an above-grade discharge area, an exhaust fan can be attached to a PVC collection pipe for drawing radon out of the soil. To maintain an effective, airtight system, a water-filled trap or reverse flow valve must be installed in the collection pipe. This water trap must be located below the frost line and must be kept filled with water. See the *Drain tile suction* drawing for additional details.

If these tiles are already present, drain tile suction is often a cost-effective approach to reducing elevated radon levels. If your home

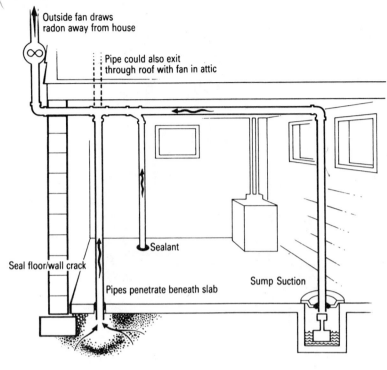

Subslab Suction

Outside fan draws radon away from house

Pipe could also exit through roof with fan in attic

Seal floor/wall crack

Pipes penetrate beneath slab

Sealant

Sump Suction

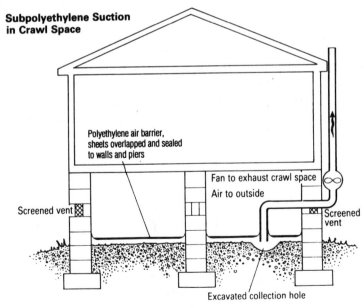

Subpolyethylene Suction in Crawl Space

Polyethylene air barrier, sheets overlapped and sealed to walls and piers

Fan to exhaust crawl space Air to outside

Screened vent

Screened vent

Excavated collection hole

Two suction techniques for under the house. (*Source: Radon Reduction Methods: A Homeowner's Guide,* third edition, EPA, July 1989.)

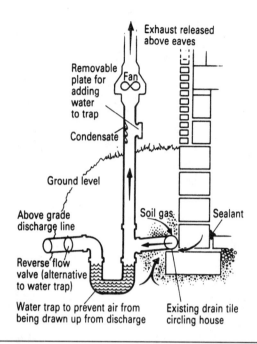

Exhaust released above eaves

Removable plate for adding water to trap

Fan

Condensate

Ground level

Above grade discharge line

Soil gas.

Sealant

Reverse flow valve (alternative to water trap)

Water trap to prevent air from being drawn up from discharge

Existing drain tile circling house

Drain tile suction. (*Source: Radon Reduction Methods: A Homeowner's Guide,* third edition, EPA, July 1989.)

already is completely looped by drain tiles, the cost of converting to a radon reducer could be as low as $100. Often, however, drain tile loops either don't go completely around the foundation of the home or some of the tiles are blocked or damaged. Unless you have a set of plans detailing drain tile locations, it's difficult to determine the exact extent or condition of the drain tile loop. Often homeowners will need to hire a professional to install or rebuild a drain tile system. Hiring a contractor to install a complete system can cost $700 to $1,500 or more.

Block wall suction. Concrete blocks used to build many basement walls contain hollow spaces that are normally connected both vertically and horizontally. Radon from the soil, entering the wall through joints, pores, and cracks, can move through these hollow spaces and enter the basement through joints and cracks on the interior side, or through uncapped openings in the top row of blocks. Block wall suction removes the radon from these spaces before it can enter the house, by creating a zone of lower pressure that reverses the direction of soil gas flow.

It is done by drilling holes into the hollow spaces in the concrete blocks and venting these holes through a plastic or sheet-metal baseboard duct around the perimeter of the basement floor. A second method involves inserting PVC pipes into the concrete walls. Fans vented to the outside are used to draw radon out of the concrete blocks. See the *Block wall suction: Two approaches* drawings for further details.

Block wall suction can be costly. Installing exhaust pipes in an unfinished basement can cost from $1,500 to $2,500; a baseboard system in an unfinished basement can cost from $2,000 to $3,000. If the basement is finished living space, cost increases. Even a do-it-yourself installation can cost $300 to $1,000 or more.

SEALING OFF RADON ENTRY ROUTES   The second major method of preventing radon entry involves closing off radon entry routes to prevent the flow of radon gas into the house. According to the EPA,

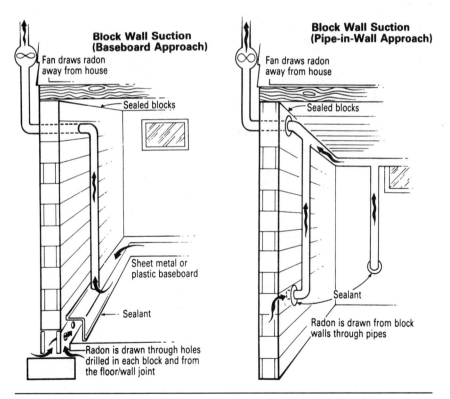

Block wall suction: Two approaches. (*Source: Radon Reduction Methods: A Homeowner's Guide*, third edition, EPA, July 1989.)

this method *should be considered an essential part of most approaches to radon reductions.*

The effectiveness of sealing is limited by our ability to identify, get to, and effectively seal major radon entry routes. Complete sealing is often impractical without incurring significant repair costs. Hard-to-reach areas that can serve as radon entry routes include: tops of block walls, spaces between block walls and exterior brick veneer, openings concealed by masonry fireplaces and chimneys, the floor above a crawl space, and below-ground areas that have been converted into living space. Nevertheless, sealing is often effective in conjunction with other radon removal methods. It's also a relatively inexpensive way to reduce radon in homes with radon levels less than 20 pCi/L.

One sealing method tested by the EPA involves placing a nylon matting under the slabs of new homes or in crawl spaces of existing homes. The matting resembles a tangle of black spaghetti with fabric backing. Its purpose is to act as an air blanket to trap the radon gas so it can be piped out. The product, known as Enkavent®, was developed by an Asheville, North Carolina, firm, Akzo Industrial Systems. The EPA tested Enkavent® in one New Jersey home that had unusually high levels of radon. After installing the spaghetti-like fabric, radon levels were reduced by 97 percent.

How to seal radon entry routes. Once radon entry routes are identified, selection of an appropriate sealant and proper preparation of the surface are critical. The drawing *Sealing radon entry routes* shows places to be sealed.

Large, exposed soil areas, such as those found in crawl spaces, can sometimes be effectively covered and sealed with a polyethylene sheet. It is also possible, if needed, to vent the air under the sheet to the outdoors by using a fan. In cases where radon levels are extremely high, a concrete slab can be poured over areas of exposed soil and then treated as a basement suitable for subslab suction.

Drainage areas such as sumps, floor drains, and perimeter drains are also significant radon entry routes. Sumps can be capped and sealed to reduce radon entry. If needed for drainage, a drain trap can be installed in the sump. Floor drains can also be rebuilt to include a trap. Traps allow the water that collects on basement floors to drain away, yet they block the entry of radon. If you use a water trap, keep its water reservoir full to maintain effectiveness.

When capping and sealing a sump, it's often advisable to install a vent so that the air trapped in the sump is exhausted to the out-

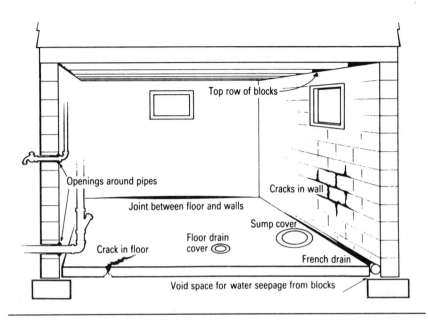

Sealing radon entry routes. (*Source: Radon Reduction Methods: A Homeowner's Guide*, third edition, EPA, July 1989.)

doors. Using a sump hole as the location for subslab suction is often very effective in reducing radon levels (see the drawing of subslab suctioning, p. 23).

Perimeter or "French" drains can be sealed with liquid urethane sealant. Cracks, joints, and utility-wire or pipe penetrations are most effectively sealed with polyurethane caulking. Field testing by the EPA has shown that latex-based caulks—even those with silicone—do not adhere well to these surfaces. Proper surface preparation is critical. Manufacturer's instructions should be followed carefully to ensure a good bond.

Paints or other pore-filling coatings are useful for large, porous surfaces such as hollow-block basement walls; however, surface cracks should first be treated with appropriate caulking material to prevent leakage. Three or more coats of latex paint probably will be required to fully seal the pores in concrete blocks; one or two coats of waterproof or epoxy paint is often equally effective.

Uncapped tops of hollow-block walls also have to be sealed to prevent radon entry. If accessible, they should be sealed with mortar or urethane foam or covered by strips of wood cemented over the openings.

Cost and maintenance. Some do-it-yourself sealing can be accomplished with materials costing $100 or less. More expensive efforts, such as the application of coatings and special membranes or films by a contractor, can cost $500 or more. The cost for a contractor to install a sump cover is about $100. If a trap is needed, costs may increase by several hundred dollars—as much as $500 for a contractor to add a water trap to a floor drain. In many cases, however, the work can be done less expensively by the homeowner.

Maintenance includes periodic inspections and resealing if a crack reopens or if settling causes any new openings to appear. If a water trap is installed, it should be refilled as necessary.

In houses with high radon levels, sealing alone probably will not reduce radon levels to below 4 pCi/L. This brings us to another method of radon mitigation: controlling the air pressure of your home.

CONTROLLING HOUSE AIR PRESSURE A primary factor contributing to the flow of radon into a home is the lower air pressure inside the house relative to the underlying soil on which it is built. This phenomenon, known as "house depressurization," is caused by what you do in your home—your activities, the number and kind of appliances you use, the design and construction features of your home, and year-round weather conditions. Exhaust fans, window, kitchen, bathroom, attic, and whole-house fans, as well as a clothes dryer, can significantly depressurize your house. Fireplaces, coal or wood stoves, central furnaces, water heaters, and other vented combustion devices can also lower the pressure within your house. To alleviate depressurization caused by forced-air heating and cooling systems, seal off any air intake registers that are in your basement or crawl space.

Experience has shown that the lower level of a house, such as a basement or crawl space, can be *pressurized* by blowing air in from either the upstairs living space or the outside. In order to reduce fan noise and vibrations in the living area, the pressurizing fan can be located on the basement floor or crawl space and connected by ducting to the outdoor air supply. To enhance the effectiveness of house pressurization, you should seal as many major openings as possible between the basement and upper floors. This means limiting the opening of doors and windows in the lower, pressurized areas.

Costs, according to the EPA, can be kept fairly low if the system is installed by the homeowner. If you hire a contractor to install a house or basement pressurization system, the cost can run from $1,000 to $2,500 and possibly more if a lot of additional sealing is needed. Running the pressurization fan would cost approximately $40 a year. However, additional heating and cooling caused by increased ventilation can cost as much as $500 a year, according to the EPA.

If house depressurization is minimized or eliminated by maintaining the air pressure of the house at higher levels, then radon entry will be reduced. In some situations, the EPA has seen reductions of up to 90 percent from systems designed to maintain positive air pressure. However, long-term experience with these techniques is limited.

NO MATTER WHAT YOU CHOOSE   No matter what you choose among the wide range of radon reduction options, the EPA recommends that you consider the following:

- Carefully inspect your home to identify potential radon entry routes such as cracks in slabs or walls, open sumps, and other house design features or appliances that may facilitate radon entry (air-consuming appliances or chimneys, for example).
- As a radon reduction method, natural house ventilation—the opening of windows alone—should be considered as only a temporary solution.
- Any system devised to reduce radon should be a permanent part of the structure and have a long life expectancy.
- A warning device should be part of all fan-assisted systems to warn of system failure.

Finding and Hiring a Professional

You will probably want to consult with experts at your state radiation office (see Directory A) to obtain whatever specific advice or assistance they can offer for your particular situation, and you may want their advice on hiring experienced radon reduction contractors. When hiring someone for radon reduction work, we cannot overemphasize the importance of carefully screening contractors and getting written bids. Ask for business references and check with your local Better Business Bureau or Chamber of Commerce. You often can save money by getting a second opinion from another contractor. You also may want to consult with your state's radiation office experts to decide if a bid is reasonable. Many states provide lists of contractors doing radon mitigation work, and some states have certification programs for radon measurement and mitigation. Some contractors even may be willing to guarantee a radon reduction to less than 4 pCi/L.

Quick Summary

Radon is an invisible, odorless, radioactive gas that can be a long-term, deadly killer. Millions of homes in the Americas and throughout the world are at risk. The risk of lung cancer from radon exposures depends on the level of radon to which one is exposed and the duration of the exposure. To determine if your home is at risk, test it for radon, but if radon is found, don't panic. Evaluate the amount of risk it presents. Use the *Radon risk evaluation chart* in this chapter (page 17). If you consider the level of risk to which your family is exposed to be unacceptable, take the necessary steps to reduce radon in your home.

ADDITIONAL RESOURCES

- "Field Comparison of Several Commercially Available Radon Detectors," an article by R. William Field and Burton C. Kross, University of Iowa Institute of Agricultural Medicine and Occupational Health, *American Journal of Public Health,* August 1990, vol. 80, no. 8, pp. 926–30.

- *A Citizen's Guide to Radon; What It Is and What to Do About It,* free from the EPA's Office of Air and Radiation, the Centers for Disease Control, and the U.S. Department of Health and Human Services. Write EPA, 401 M Street SW, Washington DC 20460, or call the EPA's Radon Hotline, 800-SOS-RADO(N) (800-767-7236).

- *Radon Reduction Methods: A Homeowner's Guide,* third edition, free booklet published by the EPA. (Write the EPA at the above address.)

- *Application of Radon Reduction Methods,* an EPA publication for homeowners seeking guidance on how to diagnose a radon problem and design a reduction method. It contains step-by-step guidance on system design, installation, and operation. (Write the EPA.)

CHAPTER 3

INDOOR AIR POLLUTION

The Enemy Within

For some pollutants, the air outside your home may be safer to breathe than the air inside your home. This was the shocking conclusion of a 10-year EPA investigation of more than 2,000 people who were exposed to a wide range of environmental pollutants in or around 12 U.S. cities.

Because most Americans spend up to 90 percent of their lives indoors (half that time in their own homes), the EPA calls the risks from indoor air pollution "among the top environmental problems" of the 1990s.

Indoor Air Pollutants Can Harm Your Health

Health effects from indoor air pollutants fall into two categories: those that are experienced immediately after exposure and those that show up years later. Long-delayed effects, such as respiratory diseases, heart disease, or cancer, can be severely debilitating or fatal. Immediate effects, which may show up after a single exposure or repeated exposures, include headaches, dizziness, fatigue, and irritation of the eyes, nose, and throat.

Many air pollutants are more concentrated inside than outside. This may be especially important for susceptible populations, such as the very young, the very old, and the chronically ill.

THOSE MOST AT RISK FROM INDOOR AIR POLLUTION   Studies indicate that as many as 15 percent of all people are hypersensitive to contaminants in the air. People most susceptible to the adverse effects of indoor air pollution, according to the EPA, are those who spend the longest periods of time indoors. These groups include the young, the elderly, and the chronically ill, especially those suffering from respiratory or cardiovascular disease.

"Typical indoor levels of pollutants can be up to 20 times higher than outdoor levels," states Ron White, senior program manager for the American Lung Association's Air Conservation and Occupational Health Program. "Children, pregnant women, the elderly, people with lung disease, and other chronic disabilities become the major victims of indoor air pollution."

How to Find Air
Pollution in Your Home

This chapter will explain the health risks from the four most widely recognized types of indoor air pollution—tobacco smoke, other hazardous combustion products (H.C.P.s), formaldehyde, and biological contaminants. We will help you diagnose potential risks in your own home and then explain what can be done to reduce these risks. (Risks from other indoor air pollutants such as asbestos, radon, lead, mercury, pesticides and other toxic household products—and the actions for assessing and reducing them—will be discussed later in this book). But first, let's test the A.Q.—the Air Quality—of your home so that you can gain a quick overview of potential air quality hazards. A totally healthy home would score a perfect 100. With that assumption, start with 100 points and subtract five points for every yes answer.

AN A.Q. (AIR QUALITY) TEST FOR YOUR HOME

1. Does your home have any unvented gas appliances? Yes [] No []
2. Do any household members smoke?   Yes [] No []
3. Do any furry pets live indoors? (Subtract five points for each pet.)   Yes [] No []
4. Are insecticides or other pesticides used indoors?   Yes [] No []
5. Are cars parked in an attached, enclosed garage? (Subtract five points for each car.)   Yes [] No []

6. Are any of the following hobbies conducted indoors: painting, woodworking, jewelry or pottery making, or model building? (Subtract five points for each.) Yes [] No []

7. Does anyone in your home use pressurized aerosol products such as hair spray and furniture polish? Yes [] No []

8. Do burner flames on gas heating or cooking appliances appear yellow instead of blue? Yes [] No []

9. Is your home insulated with materials containing urea-formaldehyde foam or asbestos? Yes [] No []

10. Are heating vents corroded or rusted? Yes [] No []

11. Does the air in your home seem stale? Yes [] No []

12. Is anyone in your family regularly experiencing symptoms such as eye, nose, and throat irritation; headaches; unusual fatigue or lethargy; shortness of breath; skin rashes; or any other symptoms of poor health of unknown origin? Yes [] No []

Did your house get a passing score of 70 or more? If you answered more than six of these questions with a yes, you may be among the millions of people with significant indoor air pollution

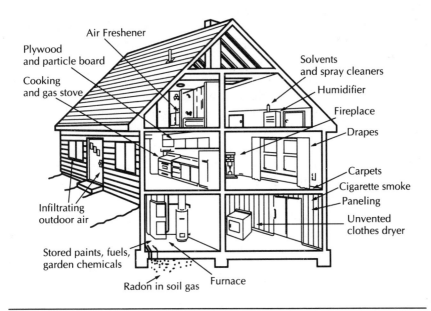

Air pollution sources in the home. (*Source: Indoor Air Pollution Research Fact Sheet*, Lawrence Berkeley Laboratory.)

problems. Of course, any yes indicates an area where you can take action to improve the air quality in your home.

The ill effects of indoor air pollution often occur when a person moves into a new residence, remodels or refurnishes a home, or treats it with pesticides. If you or any member of your family are experiencing any of the symptoms listed in question 12 of the A.Q. Test, especially if they *fade or totally go away* when you're away from the house and *return* when you're home, then try to identify potential sources of indoor air pollution.

This chapter can help you do just that: Look again at the A.Q. questions that you marked yes. Also look at the drawing *Air pollution sources in the home.* Both can serve as checklists to help you find potential sources of indoor contaminants. An important point to remember is that the relative importance of any single source depends on how much pollution it emits and how hazardous those emissions are. Now lets look at some specific indoor pollutants and the health dangers they pose.

Environmental Tobacco Smoke Pollution

Tobacco smoke is one of the most common indoor pollutants. In the United States, 50 million smokers annually smoke approximately 600 billion cigarettes, 4 billion cigars, and 11 billion pipefuls of tobacco. Since most people spend approximately 90 percent of their time indoors, this means that about 467,000 tons of tobacco are burned indoors each year. Environmental tobacco smoke (the smoke that comes from the burning end of a cigarette and smoke that is exhaled by the smoker) is a complex mixture of over 4,700 compounds, including both gases and particles. One such gas, benzene, is a known cause of leukemia in humans. EPA research has shown that "in typical homes of smokers, benzene levels on average are 50 percent higher than in homes of nonsmokers."

"The most important source of exposure (to benzene) for 50 million smokers is the mainstream smoke from their cigarettes," says Lance Wallace, Ph.D., and EPA scientist who has done trailblazing research on the "human chemical bodyburden," or the amount of chemical pollutants carried by various population groups.

THE HEALTH DANGERS POSED BY TOBACCO SMOKE   Benzene-caused leukemia is not the only risk incurred by smokers or those who live with smokers. According to reports issued by the U.S. Surgeon General and the National Academy of Sciences, tobacco smoke is definitely "a cause of disease including lung cancer *in both smokers and nonsmokers.*" Studies indicate that exposure may increase the risk of lung cancer by an average of 30 percent even for the nonsmoking spouses of smokers. Recent studies have also linked tobacco smoke to increased rates of heart disease. In fact, a January 1991 study published in *Circulation,* the journal of the American Heart Association, concludes that "passive smoking causes about 10 times as many deaths from heart disease as it does from lung cancer." Secondhand cigarette smoke kills 53,000 nonsmokers a year, including 37,000 who die from heart attacks, says Dr. Alan Blum of Houston, chairman and founder of Doctors Ought to Care, an antismoking group.

Nine million children under the age of five live in homes with at least one smoker and therefore breathe secondhand smoke every day. Young children exposed to smoke in the home are more likely to be hospitalized for bronchitis and pneumonia and to have allergies and asthma. Many pediatricians now advise parents to forbid smoking *anywhere* in the home.

"A nonsmoker is more likely to get cancer from environmental tobacco smoke than from all the hazardous outdoor air pollutants regulated by the EPA—including asbestos, arsenic, and radioactivity—combined."

EPA physicist James Replace speaking at a Harvard symposium.

HOW TO COMBAT TOBACCO SMOKE

- Open the windows, increase ventilation, or use air cleaners. But research indicates that the total removal of tobacco smoke by such measures is impossible.

- Separate smokers and nonsmokers in the same room. This may reduce, but will not eliminate, the exposure of nonsmokers to tobacco smoke because tobacco pollutants readily disperse through common air space.

- Place smokers and nonsmokers in separate rooms with separate ventilation systems that exhaust to the outdoors.

- Eliminate smoking in the building entirely.

Dangers of Hazardous Combustion Product Pollution

Hazardous combustion products (H.C.P.s) include carbon monoxide and nitrogen dioxide gases and respirable particles of various types. Sources include unvented or poorly vented kerosene, oil, coal, wood, and gas heaters, leaking chimneys and furnaces, downdrafting from wood stoves, fireplaces, and other combustion appliances, environmental tobacco smoke, and in the case of carbon monoxide—automobile exhaust from attached garages and gas appliances.

HEALTH DANGERS OF H.C.P.s Health effects of carbon monoxide poisoning include fatigue, impaired vision and coordination, headache, dizziness, confusion, and nausea. In one study, heart patients exposed to high levels of carbon monoxide suffered three times as many irregular heartbeats as those exposed to normal air.

Health effects of nitrogen dioxide include eye, nose, and throat irritation and increased respiratory infections in young children.

Respirable particles are known to cause respiratory infections, bronchitis, and lung cancer. Respirable particles include dust and any particulate matter produced by combustion, including particles produced by the burning of natural gas or heating oil. Although their sizes and chemical compositions vary, respirable particles are generally less than ten microns (one-tenth the width of a strand of baby hair) in diameter. Their light weight allows them to float in the air, where they are easily inhaled, affecting the airways and lungs, especially in people with asthma.

HOW TO PROTECT YOUR FAMILY FROM CARBON MONOXIDE AND OTHER H.C.P.s *Carbon monoxide* (CO) is an odorless, colorless gas that interferes with the ability of the blood to deliver oxygen throughout the body. Of all combustion products, CO may be the most dangerous in the short run, as it causes several hundred deaths each year. Average levels of carbon monoxide in homes without gas stoves vary from 0.5 to 5 ppm. Levels measured near properly adjusted gas stoves are often 5 to 15 ppm and near poorly adjusted stoves may be 30 ppm. Lethal CO concentrations are usually related to poor furnace maintenance; damaged chimneys, vents, and flues; improper installation of appliances; and backdrafting of furnace gases because of excess exhausts, inadequate air supply, an airtight home, or faulty auto exhaust systems. Common symptoms of CO poisoning are headache, dizziness, drowsiness, nausea, and vomiting.

Chronic exposure to low levels may contribute to cardiac disease. Note this recommendation: Have professionals check potential CO sources to make sure they are safe. But here's a safety check that any homeowner can do: The flames from a properly adjusted gas burner should be blue with only slight, yellow tips; if they are very yellow, the stove is releasing too much carbon monoxide.

The average level of *nitrogen dioxide* (NO_2) in homes without combustion appliances is about half of that outdoors. In homes with gas stoves, kerosene heaters, or unvented space heaters, indoor levels often exceed outdoor levels. So, to reduce exposure to both carbon monoxide, nitrogen dioxide, and respirable particles, take the following steps:

- Keep gas appliances properly adjusted.
- Properly vent gas space heaters and furnaces to the outdoors.
- Use the correct fuel in properly vented kerosene space heaters.
- Install and use an exhaust fan vented to the outdoors if you use a gas stove.
- Open flues when gas-fueled or wood-burning fireplaces are in use.
- Choose properly sized wood stoves that are certified to meet EPA emission standards. Make certain that doors on all wood stoves fit tightly.
- Change filters on central heating and cooling systems and air cleaners according to manufacturer's directions.
- Hire a trained professional to annually inspect, clean, and tune-up your central heating system including furnace, flues, and chimneys. Make sure all leaks are repaired.
- Do not idle your car inside the garage.

The Ubiquitous Problem
of Formaldehyde Pollution

Whenever Ben Olewine went into a certain bedroom in his New York City apartment he became sick with flu-like symptoms. "My eyes were constantly irritated and I kept sneezing, getting congested, and feeling nauseated," Olewine, a marketing consultant, told the *New York Times*. One guest who slept overnight in the bedroom became sick for two weeks.

Olewine removed everything from the room in an attempt to find the source of his symptoms. He sniffed the carpet but didn't experience any renewed symptoms. However, when he sniffed the paneling covering his wall he "sneezed like crazy." Olewine learned that he was sensitive to the formaldehyde in the adhesive used to attach the paneling.

Formaldehyde is a colorless, gaseous chemical widely used today because of its qualities as a preservative and as a bonding agent. It is one of the most important products of the chemical industry, ranking 23rd in volume of production among chemical commodities manufactured in the United States. It is found in consumer and industrial products ranging from shampoo and lipstick to toothpaste, milk cartons, car bodies, household disinfectants, kitchen cabinets, paneling, furniture, countertops, and insulation. Formaldehyde puts the "permanent" in permanent press clothing and the "strength" in wet-strength paper towels. It is widely used in pressed-wood products such as particleboard and plywood, which are widely used in furniture manufacture, home remodeling and renovation, new home construction, and mobile home construction. During the 1970s many homeowners had urea-formaldehyde foam insulation (UFFI) installed in the wall cavities of their homes as an energy conservation measure. Thus, formaldehyde is found practically everywhere.

HEALTH DANGERS OF FORMALDEHYDE EXPOSURE Formaldehyde is an irritant that at levels above 0.1 ppm can cause difficulties in breathing, nosebleeds, and irritation of the eyes, nose, and throat. People have also reported headaches, fatigue, memory loss, skin irritation, and nausea as a result of relatively low levels of formaldehyde exposure.

How many of us are at risk? No one knows for sure, but the National Academy of Sciences estimates that up to 20 percent of the population is at risk of adverse reactions from relatively low levels of exposure. While formaldehyde levels below 0.1 ppm are generally

---

National Academy of Sciences Warning

The National Academy of Sciences believes that one out of five of us are at risk of adverse reactions from exposure to relatively low levels of formaldehyde. Formaldehyde has been proven to cause cancer in animals, and several scientific groups as well as the Consumer Product Safety Commission think that it probably also causes cancer in humans.

considered safe, some hypersensitive people may react adversely to even smaller levels. For example, a small percentage of the population are so hypersensitive to formaldehyde that they react to the very low amounts found in perfumes and newsprint.

HOW TO PROTECT YOUR FAMILY FROM FORMALDEHYDE   The most unsettling aspect of formaldehyde is its potential danger to our children. A researcher in Seattle observed a high incidence of Sudden Infant Death syndrome in children who lived in formaldehyde-laden homes. If you have small children, or if you notice any of the reactions that might be due to formaldehyde, you may want to test for the presence of this chemical. Call your local health department. (See Directory A at the back of this book. It's a unique listing of the names, titles, and phone numbers of public information offices knowledgeable about air quality control issues. Most of the offices listed have experts on formaldehyde who can explain how to have your home tested or how to do it yourself.)

The good news about formaldehyde is that older homes without urea-formaldehyde foam insulation are generally found to be well below 0.1 ppm. However, in homes with significant amounts of new pressed-wood products, levels are often tested at higher than 0.3 ppm. If tests determine that the formaldehyde level in your home is 0.1 ppm or higher, you have a serious contamination problem. Don't panic. Removal of the source of formaldehyde contamination can be as simple as getting rid of the furniture that is outgasing (releasing formaldehyde molecules into the air). To further reduce formaldehyde exposure in your home, caulk or seal all routes by which formaldehyde fumes from insulation might be escaping, such as cracks around electrical outlets, baseboards, and ceilings.

BUILDING A NEW HOME   If you are having a new home built, you may want to consider instructing your contractor to avoid the use of formaldehyde-containing products, especially urea-formaldehyde foam insulation, or to use low formaldehyde-releasing pressed-wood products. Ben Olewine, the New York City apartment dweller who experienced flu-like symptoms when exposed to formaldehyde, hired a contractor to build a home using formaldehyde-free and other non-toxic materials, including solid wood and metal. Such homes usually cost about 20 percent more to build than conventionally built houses.

BUYING AN ALREADY BUILT HOME   If you are buying a relatively new home, make sure that urea-formaldehyde foam insulation (UFFI) wasn't used. (Hundreds of thousands of homes were insulated with UFFI before it was banned by the Consumer Product Safety Commission in 1982. However, this ban was later overturned by a federal court, and contractors still sometimes use it.) If you are buying an older home, you may not have to worry about UFFI or formaldehyde in general unless the home has been recently remodeled. Older homes containing UFFI should no longer have formaldehyde levels that present a significant health threat. According to the Consumer Product Safety Commission (CPSC), "after one year most UFFI homes have average formaldehyde levels below 0.1." Still, it's wise to have the home you are considering purchasing tested for formaldehyde levels before the sale goes through. If levels are high, you may want to reconsider the purchase or have steps taken to reduce formaldehyde levels.

RECOMMENDATIONS ON REDUCING FORMALDEHYDE EXPOSURE

- Before purchasing an old or a new house, ask about the formaldehyde content of pressed-wood building materials, cabinetry, and furniture. Consider purchasing metal or solid wood cabinets. Pine is popular, but be warned: Some people are allergic to pine terpenes, the fumes emitted by this wood.

- For interior work, purchase exterior-grade plywood products, which emit less formaldehyde. The exterior-grade plywood is held together by a chemically stable form of phenol formaldehyde and thus emits little formaldehyde gas. This plywood can also be substituted for particleboard in countertops and other interior uses.

- If weather permits, use air-conditioning and dehumidifiers to maintain moderate temperatures and reduce humidity levels. Such measures reduce outgasing since formaldehyde emissions are substantially increased by heat and humidity.

- To reduce outgasing in the winter, try turning down the heat. Also increase ventilation by occasionally opening doors and windows or running an exhaust fan. You and your family may have to wear sweaters and long sleeves, but an improvement in your family's health is worth the inconvenience.

The Consumer Federation of America (CFA), the nation's largest consumer advocacy organization, says: "If you suspect formaldehyde emissions in your home are too high, use vinyl wallcoverings, insulating paint, or two coats of polyurethane or varnish to seal pressed-wood surfaces . . . more importantly, ventilate your home as much as possible."

Formaldehyde Warning to Module or Mobile Home Owners

Owners of module or mobile homes may be at higher risk of formaldehyde exposure. Levels of this gaseous chemical are often higher in mobile homes because of the extensive use of pressed-wood products and the reduced ventilation in most of these dwellings. If persons living in such residences experience health problems that may be caused by formaldehyde, they should increase ventilation as much as possible and consider using the CFA procedures just mentioned for sealing pressed-wood surfaces. If health problems persist, contact the manufacturer and the dealer who sold you the home; also notify the U.S. Department of Housing and Urban Development, 451 7th Street SW, Washington DC 20410.

Biological Contaminants

Biological contaminants include bacteria and viruses, mold and mildew, animal dander and saliva, mites, cockroaches, and pollens. There are many sources for these pollutants, for example: wet or moist walls, ceilings, carpets, and furniture; poorly maintained humidifiers, dehumidifiers, and air conditioners; bedding; and household pets. Not only are household pets sources of saliva and dander but they also transmit bacteria and viruses. Even urine from rats and mice can be a problem. When cat saliva or rodent urine dries, it can become airborne and cause allergic reactions affecting the eyes, nose, and throat.

HEALTH DANGERS OF BIOLOGICAL CONTAMINANTS   Measles, rubella, smallpox, chicken pox, mumps, and respiratory infections are examples of diseases that can be transmitted by airborne viruses. Molds and mildew can cause allergies and flu-like symptoms including fatigue, nausea, shortness of breath, dizziness, fever, and eye, nose, and throat irritation. Chapter 6 on allergy and Chapter 4 on ventilation provide detailed advice on how to cope with allergy-producing substances.

Quick Summary

Indoor air pollutants come from a wide array of sources. The sources of indoor pollutants discussed in this chapter can be grouped into two general categories:

- Tobacco smoke and other combustion sources, such as fireplaces and oil, gas, kerosene, coal, or wood-burning appliances that contaminate indoor air with carbon monoxide, nitrogen dioxide, and inhalable particles
- Building materials and furnishings that give off pollutants such as formaldehyde fumes and other contaminants

There are two basic methods of combatting the sources of indoor air pollution:

- Identify and control sources of pollution to reduce and prevent indoor air contamination.
- Improve ventilation.

ADDITIONAL RESOURCES

- *The Inside Story: A Guide to Indoor Air Quality,* published by the U.S. Environmental Protection Agency and the U.S. Consumer Product Safety Commission. Write EPA Public Information Center, 401 M Street SW, Washington DC 20460, or the Consumer Product Safety Commission, Washington DC 20207.
- *Indoor Air Facts No. 5: Environmental Tobacco Smoke,* a fact sheet for the public from the EPA (same address as above item).
- *Formaldehyde: Everything You Wanted to Know but Were Afraid to Ask,* a booklet by the Consumer Federation of America. For a free copy send a self-addressed, stamped envelope to: Consumer Federation of America, 1424 16th Street NW, Washington DC 20036.
- *An Update on Formaldehyde,* a free booklet published by the U.S. Consumer Product Safety Commission. Write CPSC, Washington DC 20207.
- Additional information on formaldehyde is also available from the Formaldehyde Institute, 1330 Connecticut Ave NW, Washington DC 20036.

CHAPTER 4

REVITALIZING INDOOR AIR

Ventilation and Air Cleaning

cure

Poor air distribution throughout the home is a major factor contributing to indoor air pollution. Proper ventilation—the mixing of indoor air with outdoor air—can revitalize the air in your home and protect your health.

Ventilation Ins and Outs

It's almost as though our homes actually breathe. Outside air infiltrates through tiny cracks and holes in the walls and foundations of our houses and eventually exfiltrates through ceilings and walls. This process is similar to our own inhalation and exhalation. And just as the heart needs to pump oxygen-carrying blood to all parts of the body, fresh air needs to reach all parts of the house. How quickly air circulates depends on how tightly constructed and well-insulated your house is.

As wind passes over the roof of your home, it provides "lift," just as the air flowing over the upper surface of an airplane wing causes the aircraft to rise. That lift draws air out of the upper parts of the house, creating a steady upward flow of air through the house. Temperature differences reinforce this upward flow. Just as hot air from a fire rises up a chimney and draws cooler air in, so warm air in a house rises and works its way outside through cracks and holes in ceilings, roofs, and walls. The suction created as this warm air rises draws in replacement air through cracks and unplugged holes in the foundation or basement. This is called the *stack effect*. It is more

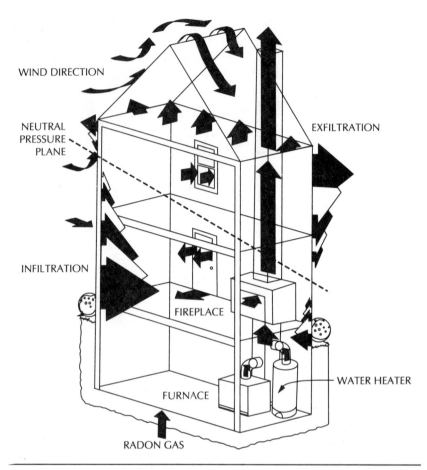

Air flow in a loose house. (Adapted and reprinted with permission from THE FAMILY HANDYMAN Magazine, Home Service Publications, Inc., an affiliate of the Reader's Digest Association, Inc., 7900 International Drive, Suite 950, Minneapolis, MN 55425 ©Copyright 1988. All Rights Reserved.)

pronounced in multilevel homes and buildings. See the drawing *Air flow in a loose house.*

Older houses are generally better ventilated than newer ones because older homes were not as tightly constructed nor as well insulated. Unfortunately, since the energy crisis of the 1970s, it has become fashionable to tighten our homes by weather-stripping, caulking, and insulating to conserve energy. This "tightening" has the effect of decreasing ventilation and increasing indoor air pollution.

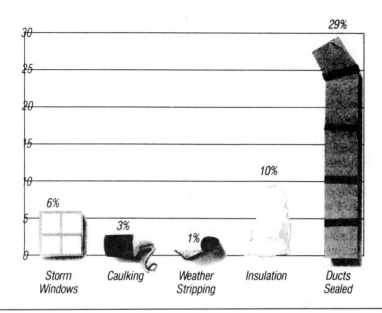

Percent reduction in air exchange rate by house-tightening measures. (*Source:* Bonneville Power Administration, Portland, Oregon.)

See the diagram *Percent reduction in air exchange rate by house-tightening measures.*

Although a "tight" house continues to "breathe," it does so at a reduced rate. Reduced ventilation increases indoor air pollution. Moisture also builds up. It enters the air from showers, baths, and other indoor water sources. Unless controlled by dehumidifiers or increased mechanical ventilation, the excess moist air tends to condense on interior surfaces, where it can breed mildew and cause wood rot, wet insulation, and peeling paint. The increased moisture also contributes to the growth of mold and mildew in the heating and air-conditioning system. The system then spreads mold spores throughout the home, causing or aggravating respiratory and other health problems.

Dampness can cause serious health problems: A Scottish study of 600 families reported in the *British Medical Journal* that an astonishingly wide range of health problems were associated with dampness. Adults reported nausea, vomiting, breathlessness, backaches, constipation, and bad nerves. When compared with children living in drier home environments, kids in damp houses had more wheezing, sore throats, runny noses, headaches, and fever. Further testing revealed that air in the damp houses contained extremely high concentrations of a wide variety of fungi.

To diagnose whether your house is susceptible to this cascade of problems, check the following:

- Do you have rooms that are particularly musty or damp? Check for a musty odor or mildew. Do your windows frequently fog up? This can be a sign of a badly ventilated home.

- Are there soot marks or black streaks on the outside of your furnace or other gas, oil, or wood-burning appliances? This is a sign of backdrafting, which occurs when a combustion appliance doesn't have enough air. Air is drawn back down the discharge vent or flue and in the process dumps combustion by-products such as soot into the home.

- Does turning on all the ventilating fans in your home (bathroom, kitchen, clothes dryer) affect the flame in your gas or oil furnace or water heater? If the flame turns yellow, produces smoke, or fails to burn steadily, you probably need better ventilation.

- Are the heating/air-conditioning vents in each room open and operating correctly? Inadequate ventilation often occurs if the air supply and return vents within rooms are blocked.

- Do you have outside-air intake vents? Every home, even in cold climates, should have air intake vents.

Evaluating Air Movement within Your Home

Experts with the American Society of Heating, Refrigerating, and Air-conditioning Engineers (ASHRAE) have studied minimum air ventilation rates necessary to dilute and remove indoor airborne contaminants and have established indoor air quality ventilation standards. ASHRAE recommends that about one-third of the air in a home be completely replaced every hour. The rate at which indoor air is replaced by outside air is called the air exchange rate, and it is measured in numbers of air changes per hour (ACH). ASHRAE recommends that a constant 0.35 ACH minimum be maintained for the whole house. That translates to replacing inside air with outside air completely about every three hours. To achieve this for a

2,000-square-foot home with eight-foot ceilings, the ventilation requirement amounts to an air flow rate of about 5,600 cubic feet per hour.

This minimum is not sufficient at all times. Ventilation requirements, such as those in the ASHRAE standards, are intended to control the products of human metabolism and other contaminants under most circumstances. The ASHRAE standard defines acceptable indoor air quality as "air in which there are no known contaminants at harmful concentrations and with which a substantial majority [usually 80 percent] of the people exposed do not express dissatisfaction." This minimum is small comfort if you are among the one-out-of-five people who are extra-sensitive.

If you or someone in your family is susceptible to indoor air pollution, ventilation rates should be increased, especially during periods of heavy use and to rooms that often need additional ventilation, such as the kitchen, bathroom, garage, and workshop. One way to do this is to install exhaust fans in these rooms, vented to the outside. Also, minimum air flow standards usually are *not* adequate when you have a full house of people. For that reason, ASHRAE also recommends an air flow rate of 15 cubic feet per minute per person. You need extra air flow if your home is besieged with strong sources of air pollution such as cigarette smoking or radon seeping from the ground.

Improving Your Home's Ventilation

There are many things you can do if you think low air-change rates in your home could be causing indoor air pollution, moisture buildup, and the resulting health problems. If your house is gasping for air, the solution is to increase the amount of outside air coming inside. Ventilate your house regularly. Leave the windows and doors open as much as possible. Let the fresh air blow through. EPA studies show that indoor air is more polluted than outside air even in urban areas. So even if your city air isn't as fresh as a country breeze, it's probably better than the stale air trapped in your home.

Often, however, the weather and home security considerations just don't permit opening windows and doors, or perhaps there isn't enough breeze to provide your home with enough air flow. In either case, you may need to install a mechanical ventilation system or, if you already have one, use it more often.

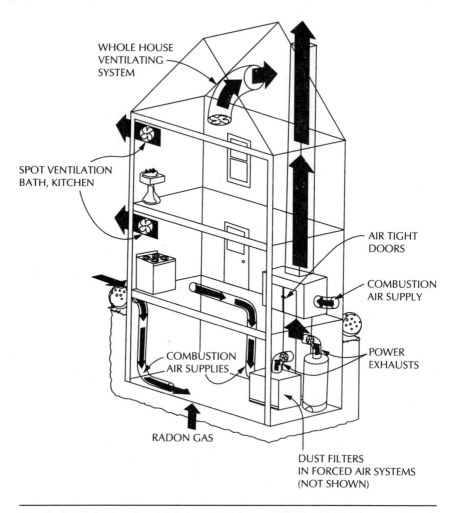

WHOLE HOUSE VENTILATING SYSTEM

SPOT VENTILATION BATH, KITCHEN

AIR TIGHT DOORS

COMBUSTION AIR SUPPLY

COMBUSTION AIR SUPPLIES

POWER EXHAUSTS

RADON GAS

DUST FILTERS IN FORCED AIR SYSTEMS (NOT SHOWN)

Ventilation solution for a tightly sealed house. (Adapted and reprinted with permission from THE FAMILY HANDYMAN Magazine, Home Service Publications, Inc., an affiliate of the Reader's Digest Association, Inc., 7900 International Drive, Suite 950, Minneapolis, MN 55425 ©Copyright 1988. All Rights Reserved.)

The drawing *Ventilation solution for a tightly sealed house* shows a two-part, general strategy for providing ideal ventilation for an absolutely tightly sealed house. First, provide appropriate air supplies *to* and *from* combustion appliances as well as exhaust from bathrooms or the kitchen. Second, provide a continuous supply of fresh air from a whole-house ventilation system, either connected to an existing forced air system or installed independently.

Window or Wall Air Conditioner Cleaning Tips

To keep your window or wall air conditioner running efficiently, do the following on a monthly basis.

- Take off the plastic, louvered front of the air conditioner and clean it with a hose or in the shower. If for some reason you can't remove the front of the unit, vacuum it instead.

- Use a vacuum-cleaner brush to remove dirt from the coils in back of the unit.

- Clean the filter by spraying water through it, washing away accumulated dirt. If the filter cannot be unclogged, replace it.

Warning: Be careful not to touch the thin aluminum fins inside the air conditioner or the coils in back of the unit, as both often have sharp edges.

EXHAUST FANS AND FRESH AIR DUCTING   The simplest ventilation system consists of bathroom exhaust fans and a kitchen range hood vented to the outside. (The EPA says that *recirculating* range hoods are inadequate for removing kitchen–generated pollutants.) Most homes are equipped with a token kitchen exhaust fan above the stove. It's relatively inexpensive to replace this with a more powerful exhaust fan. You can install a powerful exhaust fan directly into an exterior wall near the source of the exhaust gases, or, if necessary, run some ducting to the exterior wall. Although bathroom exhaust fans need to be capable of exhausting a minimum of 50 cubic feet per minute of air, kitchen exhaust fans should be capable of expelling at least 100 cfm.

Many homeowners find it more convenient to install one central exhaust fan in the basement or attic with ducts from each bathroom, the laundry room, and the kitchen. A central fan tends to be quieter because it is not in the room.

If your home has no duct system for heating or cooling, you may want to consider installing one. Fresh air can be brought into each room via a duct system dedicated to just outdoor air. One advantage to a dedicated, fresh air duct system is that outside air can be filtered before entering the house. (We'll explain more about filtering systems in the air cleaning section later in this chapter.) Although it is sometimes difficult to add ventilation without having to be creative in hiding ducting, solutions can be found. Costs vary epending on the unique features of each house. If you have a single-story home, ducts can usually run through the attic rather easily. (Be careful to seal around openings so that moisture does not escape into the attic to cause condensation problems. To prevent condensation, all duct work installed in an attic should be well insulated.) To avoid drafts, place the air supply ducts in ceilings or upper walls rather than in the floors or lower walls. Closets with louvered doors are good locations for air duct openings. This has the advantage of keeping clothes fresh and reduces mold and mildew.

FORCED-AIR VENTILATION If your home is gasping—that is, if it is without sufficient ventilation—you may have to rescue it with "artificial respiration" by using forced-air ventilation. But first consider whether your house is "tight" or "loose." Forced-air ventilation tends to be more effective in reducing pollutants in a tight rather than a loose house. (If radon is your primary indoor air pollution concern, remember that for homes with very high indoor radiation levels, ventilation should be considered only as a short-term reduction approach. For long-term safety, apply the permanent

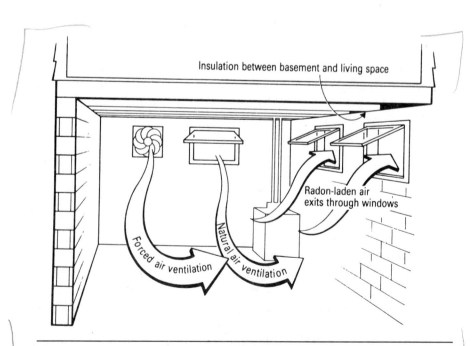

Natural and forced-air ventilation. (*Source: Radon Reduction Methods: A Homeowner's Guide*, third edition, EPA, July 1989.)

radon reduction methods explained in Chapter 2.) The drawing of a basement, *Natural and forced-air ventilation,* gives you a general idea of one approach.

Possible designs for forced-air ventilation include the installation of inward-blowing fans in windows or the use of air supply ducts to supply additional fresh air to the house. When installing a forced-air ventilation system, always place the fan so that air is blown into the house. The fan(s) should be large enough to provide at least 500 to 1,000 cfm of air depending on the size of your house and its leakiness.

The Heat Recovery Ventilator Advantage

Another way to increase ventilation and fight indoor air pollution including radon is to install a heat recovery ventilator (HRV): a device that transfers the heat of exhaust air into incoming fresh air, thereby recovering otherwise wasted heat. That explains why HRVs are also known as air-to-air heat exchangers. These devices can be installed in windows or as part of a central air system.

HRV systems have been around commercially since the late seventies, but new models are more efficient and more cost-effective than older ones. Their operating principles are simple: One fan pulls in cold, fresh air while another blows out warm, stale, house air. A heat exchange unit picks up the heat from the exhaust and transfers it to the incoming fresh air. The best units do not mix the two air streams. Most air-to-air heat exchangers come with removable air filters, and some have optional electronic or electrostatic air cleaners to keep pollen and other outdoor pollutants from entering the house.

Thad Godish, director of the Indoor Air Quality Research Laboratory at Ball State University, says HRV systems can recover 60 to 85 percent of the heat from exhaust air. The *Heat recovery ventilation* drawing shows a centrally installed system.

The primary advantages of HRV systems are reduced heating or cooling costs and greater levels of personal comfort during weather extremes. And they avoid the potential house security problem associated with leaving windows open. Dr. Godish told *Environ* magazine that "whole-house studies at Ball State show that HRV systems are particularly attractive and cost-effective in reducing formaldehyde levels in UFFI houses."

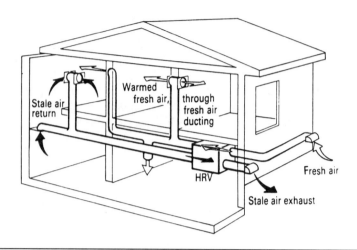

Heat recovery ventilation. In this drawing the air flows are labeled for cold weather, during which outdoor air is warmed inside the HRV. During hot weather, outside air is cooled and dehumidified. (*Source: Radon Reduction Methods: A Homeowner's Guide*, third edition, EPA, July 1989.)

Heat recovery ventilating systems are not for every home. They are most useful in climates with cold winters and/or hot, humid summers and are most effective in a tight house—one that has less than 0.5 air changes per hour (ACH). In a leaky house, airflow is diverted from the heat exchanger and escapes the energy-recovery process. For an HRV to be a reasonable option, the money saved in heating or cooling costs should be enough to offset the initial cost of the HRV in a reasonable number of years. If you live where the climate is mild, it may be less expensive to use natural or forced-air ventilation. Before a decision is made to install either a central or window HRV, the unit should be evaluated for potential energy savings, effectiveness in reducing pollution, and the overall costs compared with other options.

HRV systems can also help reduce radon. In fact, according to the EPA, an HRV system with a capacity to move 200 to 400 cubic feet per minute of air can reduce radon levels by 50 to 75 percent.

One Connecticut homeowner found radon concentrations between 4 and 10 pCi in the basement of his 20-year-old house. To flush the radon-contaminated air out of his 45 × 45 foot basement, he installed an air-to-air heat exchanger that runs continuously. His dangerous radon readings have been lowered to only 1.1 pCi/L. But

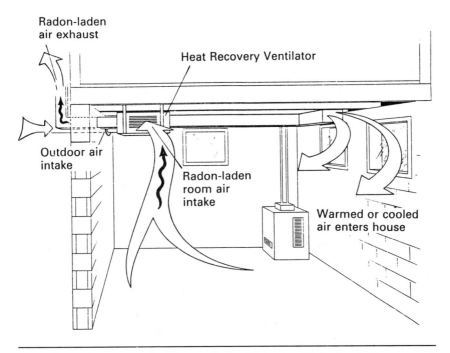

HRV for radon removal. (*Source: Radon Reduction Methods: A Homeowner's Guide*, second edition, EPA, Sept. 1987.)

don't count on HRVs if your radon levels are above 10 pCi/L. It's a technique to be used only in combination with other methods at these high levels. An HRV for radon reduction is shown in the drawing of a basement unit: *HRV for radon removal.*

HRVs are usually either ducted systems, with supply and return ducts servicing different parts of the house, or wall-mounted units similar to wall-mounted air-conditioning units. Wall-mounted units are generally less complex than ducted systems and a handy homeowner can usually install them. However, the EPA advises homeowners to hire heating and air-conditioning professionals to design and install the fully ducted systems to ensure proper installation and adjustment.

Care should be taken to position the ducting so that the fresh-air supply is located well away from the stale-air return. The cooling mechanism and fan of a ducted HRV can be installed in an inconspicuous part of the house, such as a basement or utility room. The location should be selected to make the installation of the ductwork as simple as possible.

COMPARING HRV SYSTEMS   In comparing HRV systems, consider several factors. The fans should be properly sized for maximum flow with minimum power consumption, and there should be adequate controls to prevent freezing of the coils in cold climates.

The total installed cost of a ducted HRV unit that delivers 150 to 200 cubic feet per minute of air typically ranges from about $800 to $2,500. Increasing the capacity to 300 or 400 cfm can increase the cost 25 to 50 percent, or installing a separate, second unit can double the cost.

Annual operating costs include $50 for electricity to the fan and $50 to $100 for annual servicing by a trained technician. Costs of filters vary depending on the unit.

Advice for Whatever You Choose

If you install a central system, there are several precautions to take when installing a new ventilation system, whether it's a simple central exhaust fan system, a central exhaust fan system with or without ducting, a forced-air central heating and air-conditioning system, or a heat recovery ventilator. First, ensure that combustion appliances (such as a gas- or oil-fired furnace or water heater) have their own air supply. If they don't, the new ventilation system will compete with them for air and, under some conditions, may even cause health-endangering backdrafts.

A second precaution is to ensure that the fresh air is drawn into the house from safe locations. You don't want any intake ducts to be located where they can draw in contaminated air. The outside air intake should be located a minimum of six feet from furnace, dryer, or other exhaust vents; the garage and driveway; and in Snowbelt localities it should be above the snow line.

The fresh air intake in some central systems can be controlled by either a manual or automatic volume damper. A manual damper is usually regulated by a control located next to the thermostat. With such dampers, you can choose to recirculate house air or to bring in a specific, desired amount of fresh air.

If you add a new ventilation system to your home, you should test for radon. Since more outside air will be drawn in not only through the supply ducts you have strategically installed, but also through all the tiny holes and cracks found in any house, radon may also be entering. To avoid radon and to reduce other indoor air pollution problems, experts recommend that ducts for dedicated fresh air intakes and exhaust vents be installed so as to encourage the movement of fresh air throughout the house, especially in living areas such as the recreation or family room, living room, and bedrooms. The movement of fresh air reduces levels of radon and other indoor pollutants by replacing tired indoor air with fresh, outside air.

You may also want to install ceiling fans to help keep air moving in your house or apartment.

Combatting Indoor Air Pollution with Air-Cleaning Devices

The three strategies for reducing indoor air pollutants are, in order of effectiveness, (1) controlling the sources of such pollution, (2) ventilation, and (3) air cleaning. Air-cleaning devices alone cannot ensure adequate air quality if significant pollution sources are present and ventilation is inadequate, but they may prove helpful in conjunction with the first two methods.

Air cleaners can either mechanically filter or electrostatically remove particles from the air. There are many types and sizes of cleaners on the market, ranging from relatively inexpensive tabletop models to sophisticated and expensive whole-house systems.

Although there is no universally accepted method for comparing the effectiveness of air-cleaning devices, several scientific investigators have published results using a measurement they have called a *clean air delivery rate* (CADR). This CADR number corresponds to the amount of air (in cubic feet per minute) cleaned of a specific particle. An industry source, the Association of Home Appliance Manufacturers (AHAM), has a certification program that lists the clean air delivery rates of various air cleaners according to their ability to remove dust, tobacco smoke, and pollen particles. Many portable air cleaner manufacturers are voluntary members of the AHAM program and allow their devices to be tested so they can display the AHAM seal on their products. To learn how various air cleaners came out on these tests and thus do some fast comparison shopping, you can send a self-addressed, stamped envelope with your request to: Association of Home Appliance Manufacturers, Room Air Cleaner Certification Program, 20 N Wacker Dr, Chicago IL 60606.

At the time this book went to press, portable air cleaners generally were not recommended. The effectiveness of air-cleaning devices depends on air flow rate as well as pollutant removal efficiency. Some whole-house cleaners, when connected to HVAC systems, are highly effective at particle removal. However, most portable models are much less efficient because they circulate significantly less air and aren't vented to the outdoors.

Consumer Reports magazine tested 23 portable air-cleaning units and found that only eight could effectively clean tobacco smoke and pollen-size particles from indoor air. And pollen and tobacco smoke are only two of literally hundreds of indoor air pollutants.

However, air cleaners connected to HVAC systems can significantly reduce indoor air pollution. How well an air cleaner works for you depends on a number of factors, primarily: how much air it draws through the cleaning or filtering element; how well it collects pollutants from indoors; and the type of pollutant it's up against. Pollen particles, for instance, drop out of the air very rapidly. Air filters are only effective on particles while they are suspended in the air, so an air cleaner with a high flow rate is particularly desirable if you want to reduce pollen particles.

What you can't see can hurt you. Small particles, such as those found in cigarette smoke and animal dander, settle very slowly from the air, but many heating, ventilation, and air-conditioning filters aren't effective in removing them because the small particles pass right through. Conventional filters remove particles as small as 100 microns, but they do little to screen out tobacco smoke particles, bacteria, fungi, viruses, and other particulates smaller than 100 microns. For that reason you may want to use more expensive, medium-efficiency filters, costing about $10, or HEPA (high-efficiency particulate air) filters, which cost a little more. Studies show that HEPA filters are 99.97 percent effective in removing indoor pollutants.

An alternative method is to fit your heating, ventilation, and air-conditioning system or your heat recovery ventilating system with an electronic or electrostatic filter. Such filters use positive and negative charges to remove airborne particles. The downside of electronic filters is that when they are dirty or damaged they produce ozone, itself an air pollutant that can irritate the eyes, nose, throat, and respiratory system. A better bet are the electrostatic air filters. They clean the air by using static electricity. The static charge on the filter attracts and holds airborne irritants without releasing ozone; the irritants are then washed away when the filter is cleaned.

Before buying an air cleaner or filtering system, the EPA recommends that you consider the following:

- How much air can the device handle and how much does it need to handle? Some portable air cleaners have very effective particle-removing filters, but very low air flow rates. If, for instance, an air cleaner can process only 10 cubic feet of air each minute and it is put into a typical-size room containing 1,000 cubic feet of

Air Cleaner Efficiency Rating

10%	20%	40%	60%	80%	90%
Used in window air conditioners and heating systems.	Used in air conditioners, domestic heating, and central air systems.	Used in heating and air-conditioning systems, and as prefilters to high-efficiency cleaners.	Use same as 40%, but better protection.	Generally used in hospitals and controlled areas.	Use same as 80%, but better protection.
Useful on lint.	Fairly useful on ragweed pollen.	Useful on finer airborne dust and pollen.	Useful on all pollens, the majority of particles causing smudge and stain, and coal and oil smoke particles.	Very useful on particles causing smudge and stain, and coal and oil smoke particles.	Excellent protection against all smoke particles.
Somewhat useful on ragweed pollen.	Not very useful on smoke and staining particles.	Reduce smudge and stain materially.	Partially useful on tobacco smoke particles.	Quite useful on tobacco smoke particles.	
Not very useful on smoke and staining particles.		Slightly useful on nontobacco smoke particles.			
		Not very useful on tobacco smoke particles.			

Efficiencies and uses of in-duct filtering systems. The ratings are based on ASHRAE Standard 52-76 atmospheric dust spot test. (*Source: Residential Air-Cleaning Devices: A Summary of Available Information*, EPA, February 1990.)

air, it would take about 100 minutes to process all the air in the room. Pollutants may be generated more quickly than they are removed. Similarly, a single portable unit would be of little or no use in cleaning the air of an entire house.

- What maintenance is required and what, if any, will be the decrease in performance that may occur between maintenance periods if periodic maintenance is not performed on schedule?

- What is the efficiency of the system? What percentage of particles will be removed as they go through the filtering system? ASHRAE has published two standards by which air cleaners can be compared for efficiency. The atmospheric dust spot rating, ASHRAE Standard 52-76, is used in evaluating air-cleaning units. Another indicator, Military Standard 282, is used to rate HEPA air cleaners—those with ASHRAE atmospheric dust spot ratings of about 90 percent. The chart on page 57, *Efficiencies and uses of in-duct filtering systems*, will help you to figure out what efficiency rating you want for your central filtering system.

The EPA does not endorse the use of air cleaners as a method for reducing radon because the technology of air cleaners is not effective against radon.

Looking at What the Future May Bring

A new air-conditioning/ventilation system based on a basic principle of thermodynamics (*the adiabatic process*) will probably soon become a popular means of cooling and filtering air, especially in hot, humid regions. Adiabatic change is a change during which no energy enters or leaves a closed system. The system works like this: Fresh, warm outside air is sucked through a heat exchanger where it sheds heat by being passed through a salty mist. The outside air is dried and cooled by the water-absorbing action of the concentrated salt solution. The now cooled and dried air then flows through water sprayers, which remove dust, pollen, and other particulates, before it enters the living environment. The clean, cool air moves at a rate of about four miles per hour (the average speed of a person walking) and pushes the polluted, inside air to the outside through an exhaust system.

"The system will exchange the total volume of air inside a 1,500-foot home three to four times every hour," says James Beckman,

Ph.D., an Arizona State University professor, who predicts that adiabatic coolers will replace standard air-conditioning systems within ten years. He describes them as follows:

> Standard air conditioners use a compressor and refrigerants to cool a volume of air, then continually recirculate that air complete with its load of particulates, odors, and allergens. Most air-conditioning systems use chlorofluorocarbon (CFC)-based refrigerants, but they are on the way out because CFCs have been shown to harm the environment. The adiabatic process doesn't use noisy, energy-consuming compressors, nor does it need CFCs. It consists of several fans and pulleys plus the special salt mist mechanisms. The system can deliver two tons of cooling capacity while using 50 to 60 percent less energy than typical air-conditioning systems. Besides cooling the home, it provides healthy, allergen-free air.

Quick Summary

Just as inadequate blood circulation is bad for the health of our bodies, so is inadequate air circulation bad for our homes. If any telltale signs appear, such as musty odors, soot, or yellow flames in your gas-fired appliances, you should take immediate steps to improve the flow of fresh air into your home. When considering ventilation and air-cleaning options there are many factors to consider, including the volume of air in your home, the strength of pollutants, the "tightness" of your house, and the effectiveness of the ventilation and/or air-cleaning system you are considering. Heat recovery ventilators and electrostatic filters are excellent solutions to many indoor air ventilation and cleaning problems.

ADDITIONAL RESOURCES

- *Environ: A Magazine for Ecologic Living and Health,* published quarterly; subscription is $15 for four issues. Address: *Environ,* P.O. Box 2204, Fort Collins CO 80522.

- For information regarding HRV systems write: Renewable Energy Information, P.O. Box 8900, Silver Spring MD 20907. They will send you a U.S. Department of Energy fact sheet entitled *Air-to-Air Heat Exchangers.*

- Before buying a mechanical ventilation system, you may want to discuss your home's unique needs with local experts. You can look in the phone book's yellow pages under "Engineers" or write the American Society of Heating, Refrigerating, and Air-conditioning Engineers (ASHRAE) for the address of the local ASHRAE organization. Write: ASHRAE, 1791 Tullie Cir NE, Atlanta GA 30329.

- For further information on standards for in-duct air cleaners, contact: Air-conditioning and Refrigeration Institute (ARI), 1501 Wilson Blvd, 6th Floor, Arlington VA 22209.

- For an in-depth analysis of air cleaners, write for the EPA document, *Residential Air-Cleaning Devices: A Summary of Available Information.* Contact: Public Information Center, U.S. Environmental Protection Agency, Mail Code PM-211B, 401 M Street SW, Washington DC 20460.

CHAPTER 5

ASBESTOS

A Hidden Killer In Your Home?

In 1988 42-year-old Marvin Selph with his wife, Carol, 40, and their three children abandoned their Jasper, Florida home, leaving behind almost everything they owned. Workmen earlier had cut openings for air-conditioning and heating ductwork in the walls of their home and discovered that the wallboard was made largely of asbestos. When fine, gray particles of asbestos began settling on their clothing and personal belongings, the Selph family fled their home. Their escape, while a drastic action, may have saved their lives. Asbestos exposure, over time, can kill. Asbestos could be a hidden danger in your home too.

Asbestos is a term describing a family of fibrous minerals commonly used in a variety of construction materials through the years because it is strong, durable, resists fire, and is an efficient insulator against heat or cold. Although banned in the 1970s as a spray-on fire retardant and as a wrapping for water pipes, asbestos alone—or in combination with other materials—could have been used in your house in flooring, walls, and ceiling tiles, exterior housing shingles, and electrical systems before 1989 when it was banned by the EPA for almost all commercial applications.

Health Dangers of Asbestos

Asbestos causes no immediate health effects or symptoms, but in the long run it can cause chest and abdominal cancers and lung diseases. We've known that asbestos is hazardous since the first century A.D. when Pliny Secundus, a Roman, wrote about the shortness of breath experienced by slaves who worked with asbestos. Centuries later, as commercial production of asbestos began in Europe, case reports appeared as early as 1894 describing asbestos fiber inhalation in the workplace as "injurious to the lung." In 1924 an English physician named Cook described the presence of "curious bodies" in the lungs of asbestos workers.

Modern-day doctors have described in detail how inhaled asbestos particles attach to the lining of the lungs, where over time they can cause an irreversible lung disease called asbestosis, lung cancer, or a rare cancer of the chest and abdominal linings called mesothelioma. The risk for smokers who are exposed to high levels of asbestos is even higher than that for nonsmokers.

Soft, friable (easily crumbled) asbestos materials have the greatest potential for causing health problems. Asbestos materials can start to crumble because of age, accidental damage, or as a result of normal cleaning, construction, or remodeling activities. After a crumbling asbestos material has been disturbed, the asbestos fibers—because they are so small and light—can remain in the air for hours and are usually invisible. Even after they settle on a surface, they are dangerous because they can become airborne again. If inhaled or swallowed, they can accumulate in the lungs and elsewhere in the body and, like tiny time bombs, cause health difficulties decades later. (Although even one asbestos fiber could theoretically cause cancer, one's risk is directly related to the amount and duration of exposure.)

SIGNS AND SYMPTOMS OF ASBESTOS EXPOSURE If you or your family members have been subjected to prolonged exposure to significant amounts of asbestos dust or airborne fibers *in the home or on the job,* you should see a physician specializing in lung diseases or occupational medicine. The key words here are "prolonged exposure." Low-level exposure usually doesn't result in disease. Some experts believe that the estimated risk of premature death from asbestos exposure is one in 100,000 or less. So, if you or members of your family have been exposed to small amounts of asbestos on isolated occasions, don't panic. The odds are in your favor.

If, though, like Marvin Selph's family you are at risk of being exposed to large amounts of airborne asbestos dust or fibers for a long period of time, you should take action to eliminate your exposure. And if you have already been exposed to significant amounts of asbestos dust or airborne fibers for a long duration, whether the exposure was in the home or on the job, be vigilant for symptoms listed in the box titled Symptoms of Asbestos-Caused Disease.

Experts predict that by the end of the century as many as 200,000 American deaths will have been caused by asbestos-related diseases. Court cases involving asbestos injuries, most resulting from prolonged occupational exposure, have clogged federal courts and forced major asbestos-mining companies into bankruptcy.

Symptoms of Asbestos-Caused Disease

If any of the following symptoms develop, schedule an examination by your doctor without delay:

- Shortness of breath
- A cough, change in cough pattern, or persistent respiratory illness
- Pain in the chest or abdomen
- Difficulty in swallowing or prolonged hoarseness
- Significant weight loss

Identifying Materials
That Contain Asbestos

Although it's true that both the EPA and the Consumer Product Safety Commission (CPSC) have banned many asbestos products, the CPSC believes that asbestos is still present in 75 percent of all American homes. Elevated levels of the dangerous fiber tend to occur in older homes where asbestos-containing materials such as insulation, fireproofing, or acoustical materials are damaged, deteriorated, or disturbed. It can be present in newer homes if dry wall construction was used. Also patching, spackling, and joint compounds may contain asbestos.

Look for friable asbestos around coverings of old furnaces and water pipes and as the insulation in crawlspaces and attics. In the past, water pipes were often wrapped with asbestos insulation. If your pipes are insulated with cloth-wrapped, circular cardboard with a whitish color, chances are it's asbestos. Don't panic. Asbestos pipe insulation that is perfectly wrapped and not crumbling should be left alone. If the insulation is crumbling, it should be removed, but never try to remove it yourself. Get professional help.

Don't touch any loose asbestos. According to some experts, even small amounts of airborne asbestos can theoretically cause health problems years down the road. Extreme caution is needed in handling any material suspected of containing asbestos. If the suspected material is likely to be banged, rubbed, taken apart, or otherwise handled, hire a contractor trained in asbestos control techniques. The type of asbestos professional you hire will depend on the type of asbestos product and what needs to be done to correct the problem.

Refer to the drawing of the house *Locating asbestos*; the numbers in the drawing match the numbers in the following list of common locations and products that in the past have contained asbestos and the conditions that may release asbestos fibers.

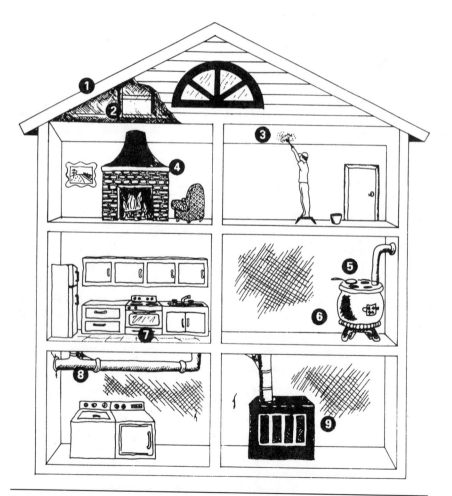

Locating asbestos. (*Source:* American Lung Association.)

1. Twenty years ago *cement roofing and siding* were often made with asbestos, but it's unlikely these products will release fibers unless sawed, drilled, or cut.

2. Houses built between 1930 and 1950 may have asbestos as *insulation*.

3. Homes built or renovated between 1945 and 1978 may have *ceilings or walls covered with textured paint* containing asbestos. Asbestos soundproofing or decorative material sprayed on walls and ceilings can release fibers when these materials are loose, crumbly, or water-damaged. In addition, *patching and joint compounds* for walls and ceilings sometimes contained asbestos. Sanding, scraping, or drilling through any of these surfaces may release asbestos.

4. *Artificial ashes and embers,* which used to be sold for use in gas fireplaces, may contain asbestos.

5. Fireproof *gloves,* stove-top *pads,* some ironing board covers, and certain hairdryers contained asbestos. If you have such items, they will ultimately deteriorate and pose a danger to your health if you keep them. Dispose of these items before they start shedding fibers. If they have started to deteriorate, carefully put them into a plastic garbage sack, seal it, and label it as containing asbestos. If your city has a hazardous waste disposal site, drop it off there. If not, follow the instructions in Chapter 10 on handling toxic products.

6. *Cement sheet, millboard, and paper* used as insulation around furnaces and wood-burning stoves often contain asbestos. Repairing or moving these appliances or cutting, tearing, sanding, drilling, or sawing the insulation can release asbestos fibers.

7. Unless you know for a fact that a synthetic *floor* does not contain asbestos, assume it does. Asbestos was still being added to some vinyl floor tiles and to the *backing or adhesive* of vinyl sheet flooring, until 1986. Assume that vinyl, asphalt, and rubber tiles are frequently sources of asbestos fibers. Sanding or scraping the tiles, or sanding or scraping the backing of sheet flooring, can release asbestos fibers into the air.

8. Hot-water and steam *pipes* as well as boiler and furnace ducts, in homes built between 1920 and 1972, were often insulated with asbestos wrap or sealed with asbestos paper tape. These materials, if damaged, repaired, or removed improperly can release asbestos fibers into the air that you and your family breathe.

9. Door *gaskets* in furnaces, wood stoves, and coal stoves may contain asbestos. Worn seals can release asbestos fibers during use.

List of Suspect Asbestos-Containing Materials

- Cement pipes, cement wallboard, and cement siding
- Vinyl wall coverings
- Asphalt and vinyl floor tile
- Vinyl sheet flooring
- Flooring backing
- Ceiling tile and lay-in panels
- Adhesive compounds for floor, carpet, or ceiling tile
- Acoustical and decorative plaster
- Textured paints and coatings
- Spray-applied or blown-in insulation
- Fireproofing materials
- Heating and electrical ducts and flexible fabric connections in ventilation ducts
- Pipe insulation
- Electrical wiring insulation
- Wallboard
- Roofing shingles and roof felt
- Caulking, putties, and spackling compounds

Asbestos may be hidden in many different building materials. Unless it is labeled, there is usually no way of telling if a material contains asbestos simply by looking at it. If you have a material, such as acoustical tile, that is damaged or that you plan to cut through or sand during remodeling, you should treat it as if it contained asbestos or have it sampled and analyzed by a qualified professional.

Don't sample possible asbestos materials yourself. If done incorrectly, sampling can be more hazardous than leaving the material alone.

Help from Asbestos Professionals

Most home repair or remodeling contractors do not have the required tools, training, experience, or equipment to work safely with asbestos or to remove it from the home. However, there is a growing band of asbestos professionals who *can* conduct home inspections, take samples of suspected material, assess its condition, and advise about what corrective action might or might not need to be taken. The federal government and some state governments have training courses and certification programs for asbestos professionals. To locate such a professional, contact your state asbestos expert (see Directory A); check with your local air pollution control board, your state or local health department, or your EPA regional office (see Directory B). Once you contact asbestos professionals, ask them to document their completion of federal or state-approved training.

SAFETY GUIDELINES WHEN ASBESTOS SAMPLES ARE TAKEN   The professional you hire, to avoid contaminating your home and to protect your family, should at a minimum observe the following procedures when taking a sample.

- Shut down the heating, cooling, and ventilation systems to minimize the spread of any inadvertently released asbestos fibers.
- Make sure no one else is in the room when sampling is done.
- Spray the area where the sample is being taken with a fine mist of water laced with a few drops of detergent to reduce the release of asbestos fibers.
- Wear disposable gloves and other protective clothing.
- Place a plastic sheet under the area to be sampled.
- Take care not to disturb the material any more than is needed to take a small sample.
- Put the sample into a clean plastic or glass vial or a strong plastic bag, and tightly seal it. The sample should be labeled with an identification number, a date, and information as to where and from what the sample was taken.
- Clean up with a damp paper towel or other absorbent materials anything on the outside of the container or around the sampled area.
- The wipe-up materials should be placed on the plastic sheet, which should then be carefully rolled up and sealed with tape. It should be sealed in a plastic bag with a large warning label attached informing sanitation workers that the bag contains asbestos cleanup materials.

- The sampled area should be sealed with duct tape to prevent fiber release.

- The sample should be sent to an EPA-approved laboratory for analysis. You can check whether the laboratory is EPA-certified by contacting the National Institute for Standards and Technology (NIST). Write: Laboratory Accreditation Administration—NIST, Gaithersburg MD 20899; or call 301-975-4016.

Asbestos Do's and Don'ts for the Homeowner

- *Don't* use abrasive pads or power strippers to strip wax from asbestos flooring.

- *Don't* try to work with asbestos flooring or its backing yourself. When asbestos flooring needs replacing, install new floor covering over it.

- *Don't* dust, sweep, or vacuum debris that may contain asbestos, but also take care not to track it through the house. Have it cleaned with a wet mop or special equipment used by asbestos mitigation experts. (The wet mop should be thrown away or at least thoroughly cleaned after use.)

- *Do* have suspect materials tested by asbestos professionals to see if they contain asbestos.

- *Do,* after checking references and credentials, hire asbestos professionals—if possible with a firm other than the one that tested your home—to seal, enclose, or remove the asbestos.

Corrective Action

If you find that you have an asbestos material in your home and it is cracking or flaking asbestos, you should get expert help. Call a contractor experienced in asbestos control rather than trying to correct the problem yourself. The CPSC and the EPA recommend that you *not* hire the same firm that diagnosed your home's asbestos problem to correct it because of possible conflicts of interest. Before hiring the professional asbestos abatement contractor, check the firm's credentials carefully. Make sure they are trained, experienced, reputable, and accredited. Check with state or federal accreditation agencies and the Better Business Bureau, and ask for references from previous clients. Find out if these clients were satisfied. Get cost estimates from several reputable firms, and hire one only after discussion of the unique problems in your home and after you have a good understanding of the steps that contractor will take. There are four types of corrective actions: encapsulation, enclosure, repair, and removal.

Encapsulation involves a professional treating the material with a sealant such as epoxy that either binds the asbestos fibers together or coats the material so that the fibers are not released.

Enclosure involves covering or placing something over and/or around the asbestos material to prevent the release of fibers. For instance, exposed insulated piping may be covered with a protective wrap or "jacket."

Repair activities may be feasible on small areas of asbestos-containing materials. Asbestos professionals may, for instance, be able to repair an isolated area of crumbling asbestos by using the "glove bag" technique. This method involves being able to put a plastic bag over the asbestos area and doing the repair while using gloves. Any asbestos fibers dislodged during the procedure settle in the plastic bag. (Warning: This procedure is for asbestos professionals only.)

The fourth option, *removal,* should be the option of last resort. It is the most costly, and studies show that the process of removing the asbestos may actually increase the health risk, because fibers almost inevitably get into the air and are spread through the house. Once contaminated, ridding a house of asbestos fibers can be extremely expensive. Make sure your asbestos professional knows how to work under a negative air-pressure containment field to reduce the spread of asbestos fibers.

Which approach is best? Repair of small areas is often least costly. Areas that are not readily accessible to humans, such as piping in crawl spaces, are often enclosed. Areas not easily enclosed are often encapsulated. Costs vary, according to the difficulty and amount of work. Many firms charge from $70 to $100 or more per hour.

However, the EPA and the American Lung Association caution that asbestos removal is often *not* a homeowner's best course of action. *There is a fifth option—often the best.* Since asbestos fibers are harmless unless breathed, and since even good removal jobs may temporarily raise fiber levels in the air, the best thing to do with asbestos material, in good condition, is to *leave it alone.* In fact, an improper removal can create a dangerous situation where none previously existed.

Quick Summary

The inhalation of asbestos fibers can have serious health consequences that may not appear for years. That explains why it is important to inspect your home for asbestos materials, especially where there are signs of crumbling. During your inspection, take every precaution possible to avoid damaging materials that might contain asbestos. If you identify undamaged asbestos materials in your home, leave them alone. If in doubt as to whether the material is asbestos, don't saw, sand, scrape, or drill holes in the material yourself. Have asbestos sampling, repair, and, if necessary, removal done by people properly trained and qualified in handling this dangerous mineral.

ADDITIONAL RESOURCES

- The EPA maintains an asbestos hotline to answer questions about asbestos, including whether your state has a training and certification program for asbestos removal contractors. Phone 202-554-1404 from 8:30 A.M. to 5:00 P.M. EST.

- Along with the American Lung Association and the Consumer Product Safety Commission (CPSC), the EPA has a free, informative booklet for homeowners concerned about asbestos. Send a postcard to: Asbestos in the Home, Washington DC 20207. That's the complete address.

- For suggestions on controlling asbestos exposure inside schools and other buildings (some of the material is pertinent to homeowners), write for *Guidance for Controlling Asbestos-Containing Materials in Buildings* and *Managing Asbestos In Place: A Building Owner's Guide to Operations and Maintenance Programs for Asbestos-Containing Materials*. Address your request to: Environmental Assistance Division—EPA, TS-799, 401 M Street SW, Washington DC 20460; or call the Asbestos Hotline 202-554-1404.

- The Food and Drug Administration (FDA) is concerned about asbestos contamination of food, drugs, and cosmetics. For answers to questions on these topics write: Consumer Inquiries, FDA, 5600 Fishers LN, HFE-88, Rockville MD 20857.

- For questions about the potential hazards of asbestos in commercial products, write to the CPSC at 5401 Westbard Ave, Bethesda MD 20207. The CPSC also has a toll-free number providing general information on current consumer matters. Call 800-638-CPSC.

CHAPTER 6

THINGS YOU BREATHE, EAT, AND TOUCH

How to Allergy-Proof Your House

The Bible refers to a plague of boils that occurred in Egypt thousands of years ago. Some scientists now believe that it was actually a plague of skin allergies caused by tiny particles of ash landing on the skin. The ash was from the furnaces in use at that time. Allergies have been with us through the ages, but there have never been as many factors to cause them as we have with us today.

We are surrounded by a sea of substances that can cause allergies. Technology has brought thousands of new chemicals into the home, the garden, and even the playpen. From the moment you put on your shoes in the morning until you crawl under a blanket at night you are in contact with hundreds of substances in your own private sea of stuff. Any one of them could cause you trouble.

For instance, in California a woman's eyes swelled nearly shut, red blotches covered her skin, and itchy hives broke out over her arms and back. By the time she reached a doctor, she could barely breathe. In Kansas, a man sneezes, his nose drips, his eyes water and itch, his ears and throat itch inside. He struggles to get a few hours of sleep each night, but scarcely has the energy to drag himself out of bed to go to work. He has been this way for months. A housewife in Des Moines gets a scaly red rash every summer, and at other times gets frequent pounding headaches. A ten-year-old boy in Tucson constantly sniffs and coughs. He usually has his mouth hanging open because he can't breathe through his nose. He gets ear infections every two months or so. Their troubles are all caused by allergies to something in their homes.

Symptoms

If you have some illness that simply won't go away despite treatment, it may be due to an allergy, and you may be able to get rid of it by allergy-proofing your life. Suspect an allergy if you have: frequent sneezing, a snuffly or runny nose, itching of the palate and ear passages, red, itchy eyes, "sinus trouble," asthma, hives or rashes, frequent headaches, frequent earaches, coughing, or frequent gastrointestinal problems. Many of these symptoms can be due to other pollutants that we have discussed, but they are particularly indicative of an allergy.

Holiday Headache

A middle-aged man had recurrent, severe headaches on Thanksgiving, Christmas, and New Year's Day. One doctor thought he drank too much alcohol on the holidays. A psychiatrist thought it was because his mother-in-law always visited. An allergist found that he was allergic to penicillin; his holiday turkeys came from a state where they were fed on a mash containing penicillin.

Allergies can cause many symptoms and can mimic many diseases, leaving doctors and patients baffled because nothing seems to cure them. The woman who is always tired, the baby who doubles up and screams with colic, the child who has ear infections or colds over and over or who is inattentive in school, the man or woman who has frequent pounding headaches, or the person who has diarrhea, stomachache, gas pains: All may have trouble caused by allergies.

Christmas Trees

"Many people find themselves plagued during the holiday season with allergy symptoms: runny nose, watery eyes, sneezing, and coughing. Often they do not realize that a Christmas tree may be the source of their misery."

Dr. Timothy Sullivan, chief of allergy, University of Texas Southwestern Medical Center.

Even frequent, unexplained depression or other mental problems can sometimes be caused by allergies. Red and yellow dyes in foods and medicines, for example, have sometimes been reported as the cause of mental confusion, depression, delusions, crying spells, and other symptoms thought to be mental illness.

In an infant or young child there may be colic, diarrhea, spitting up a large amount of formula, or a persistent cough. The child may have extreme likes and dislikes in foods, may be cranky or irritable, or may have what allergists call "the allergic salute"—constantly pushing the nose up or sideways to get more air. This repeated upward rubbing can cause a permanent crease across the bridge of the nose that an allergist can spot whenever an allergic patient comes into the office.

In infants and very young children the symptoms are sometimes masked. Children may simply have ear stuffiness and hearing impairment with none of the other adult symptoms, or they may have only prolonged nasal stuffiness or mild "pinkeye," only later developing into adult-type symptoms. A child who has many colds during the year—who is "susceptible to colds"—is more than likely a child with a respiratory allergy. Doctors call it *perennial allergic rhinitis*. The condition comes and goes, and parents usually figure the child is just having another cold when it is really an allergy. The child may have a partial hearing loss or may sometimes say his head feels heavy, blocked, or full; or the child may feel or hear fluid in the ear when turning the head. Sometimes neither parent nor child realizes there is a hearing loss, so that the child may be considered inattentive or slow in understanding or even disobedient. If you notice any of these signs in your child, take the child to a physician for a thorough examination and discuss the problems and your theories with the doctor.

"About one in six Americans suffer from allergies and/or asthma."

National Center for Health Statistics.

"Deaths from asthma have more than doubled in this decade... children lose more than 150 million school days annually because of asthma and hayfever, adults more than 10 million work days a year."

The Asthma and Allergy Foundation of America.

> "A steady, worldwide increase in deaths from asthma has left the international medical community bewildered."
>
> *1990 World Conference on Lung Health, Boston.*

Tracking Down the Clues

There are three major categories of things that can cause allergies:

1. Things you breathe (dust, chemical vapors, animal dander, feathers, pollen, molds)
2. Things you eat or drink (foods, drinks, medicines)
3. Things you touch (fabrics, plants, metals, woods, plastics, cosmetics, soaps)

It's not always easy to trace the source. The same troublemaker in different people can cause entirely different symptoms. One person's allergic reaction to eating chocolate, for example, may be swollen eyes the next morning; another person may get hives; another might have diarrhea, and another a severe headache.

Nor is there any relationship between how the troublemaker gets into your body and what symptoms it causes. Something you breathe may cause a skin rash, whereas something you eat may cause breathing difficulties and not even affect your digestive system. The only way you can understand your particular problem is to ferret out the clues in your own situation.

It's important to work with your doctor, because any of these symptoms can also be caused by other things. Coughing and shortness of breath could be due to allergy, but could also be due to emphysema, cancer, an infection, or heart trouble. Or a cough can be a nervous habit.

A physician who specializes in allergy will be able to help you by analyzing what you tell him or her about the patterns of your symptoms, such as when and where and how they occur, and allergists can often determine the causes of your allergies with skin and other tests. Even though your doctor may be Sherlock Holmes, *you'll* need to be Dr. Watson: Much of the work in finding clues will be up to you.

If your child has the allergy, let him or her be a detective too. Explain that you are trying to find out what is bothering him and causing the itching or sneezing. Ask if he has any ideas when it is worst or what might cause it. Your child may astonish you with some very observant remarks and good clues.

Ask yourself if there has been any time pattern in the appearance of symptoms—can they be related to a pollen season or to spring housecleaning? Do the symptoms persist for long periods, or do they occur over and over? Are they related to any special place? Do symptoms appear at home but not away? Can specific foods be associated with the gastrointestinal distress, or with the rash?

Think first about some of the most common causes of allergies. Among airborne allergens, for example, the most common trouble-makers include animal dander, ragweed, grass pollens, tree pollens, molds, and dust.

To find out if one of these is likely to be causing your trouble, think about when the symptoms occur. Do they occur in the spring, summer, fall, or year-round? Do you generally have the symptoms during a specific time of day or night? Do you have symptoms only in certain rooms? Or after you have done certain things? If sneezing and runny nose come in August and September, you are probably allergic to ragweed pollen. If you sneeze in the spring, you are probably allergic to the tree pollens. If you sneeze during the summer, it is likely to be grass pollens.

"Since new chemicals that can serve as potent sensitizers are continually coming into use, the flow of patients can only be expected to continue."

Drs. Raymond G. Slavin and Deanna F. Ducomb, of St. Louis University School of Medicine, in Hospital Practice.

But it's not always pollen. One family found their baby was fine except when she crawled around on the floor; then her nose would start dripping and she would begin to cough. The cause: the pad under the living room carpeting. Another baby had symptoms when in bed. His troublemaker: the comforter his grandmother had bought.

Sometimes the cause is not easy to find. A few years ago the visits for asthma to asthma clinics in four New York City hospitals abruptly increased. The increase in the number of asthma visits occurred on the same days at all four hospitals in the fall. There was no increase in pollens or molds, but the increased visits did coincide with the onset of early cold spells and the beginning of the heating season. The people had not cleaned their filters when they turned their furnaces on.

The Case of a Wrong Diagnosis
A housewife was sick nearly all her life with wheezing, headaches, even blackouts. She often staggered about, was depressed, and had muscle and joint pain. The only time she seemed well was when she was outside. She had several attacks in her kitchen that her family doctor diagnosed as epilepsy. After years of suffering it was determined that she was allergic to the gas in her cooking stove and furnace.

Could you be allergic to your house? Here are some typical allergy-producing places to check:

- Bedroom: The rug may have a moldy pad. You may be allergic to feather pillows.
- Den: A favorite old chair may have down cushions.
- Cellar or attic: A damp cellar may mean mold, and an unused attic means dust.
- Friend's home: Perhaps there is a dog or a parakeet in a house where you frequently visit.
- Weekend cottage in the country: There may be old feather pillows and dust, or the previous owner may have housed chickens and horses in the barn.
- Playground: Ragweed or other pollen-producing plants may be nearby.
- Home improvements: There may be paint or varnish fumes, or you may be in contact with cleaning solutions or dust.

You may find it helpful to keep a notebook or diary to keep track of your symptoms and what you were doing when they occurred.

"Dust-proofing measures are particularly effective when applied to the bedroom, and can result in substantial health benefits to the allergic patient." *American Academy of Allergy and Immunology.*

If You Are Allergic to Pollen

- Stay in the house with windows closed, especially between 5:00 and 10:00 A.M. when pollen levels are usually highest or when it's windy, and keep windows closed at night when you sleep.
- Wear glasses or sunglasses outdoors to protect your eyes from pollen.
- Have your lawn mowed short to avoid pollen release from the grass.
- If you have been exposed to pollen, take a shower and shampoo your hair when you come indoors. (When you're outdoors, your hair collects and holds pollen.)
- Keep your hands away from your eyes.
- Avoid handling objects covered with dust, such as books, boxes, or clothing that have been stored.
- If you are allergic to any foods, even mildly, avoid them during the pollen season, because ingesting them will add to your symptoms, even though they may not give you much trouble the rest of the year. Also avoid alcohol during hayfever times.
- During the pollen season, take extra vitamin C, which has been shown to help alleviate many of the symptoms.
- Avoid cigarette smoke.
- If you have chest congestion or wheezing, it often helps to use a vaporizer, to turn on the hot water in the shower and inhale the steam, or to drink a hot cup of coffee or tea (caffeine and heat both help relax bronchial spasms).

If it is only seasonal pollen you are allergic to, you may find that the simplest thing to do is to take a vacation during that season, going to a part of the world where that pollen doesn't exist. For example, ragweed pollen is largely absent in deserts, on high mountains, or in far northern woods; or you can get away on a cruise. Unfortunately, as formerly pollen-free areas become populated and developed, ragweed begins to grow there, so that many places that were pollen-free for hayfever holidays ten or twenty years ago are no longer satisfactory.

If you think that moving to a new climate is the answer for you, experts suggest that you don't sell your house and make a permanent move right away. If possible, try the new location out

Each of the three pollen-producing groups (trees, grasses, and weeds) has its own season, which differs from region to region across the United States. Here is a chart that pinpoints the worst pollen months for each region.

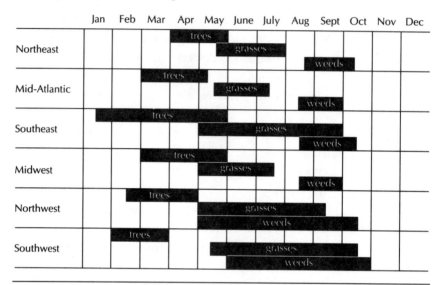

Peak pollen periods in the United States. (*Source:* Allergy Information Center.)

for at least a year to see how much benefit you have before you make a permanent move. Because different pollens may complicate the problem of your finding a suitable haven, you should always consult your physician about your particular allergy. (See the chart *Peak pollen periods in the United States.*)

Dust Allergy

If you often feel like you're catching a cold on cleaning day or if you sneeze and sniffle when you go through old things in the attic, change the draperies, or take rugs for cleaning, you are probably allergic to dust. Various studies to determine the incidence of allergy to dust show that anywhere from 45 to 80 percent of hayfever and asthma patients are sensitive to it. The older dust becomes, the more potent it is in causing allergic symptoms. Many people think that they sneeze only from the tickle of the dust balls in the nose, but usually the sneezing is an allergic reaction of the entire body.

Be suspicious of allergy to house dust if (1) your symptoms increase when you dust, clean, or carry out other household duties or (2) your symptoms increase when you turn on the heating units as the weather turns cold. Keeping your house dust-free is of utmost importance.

INSECT DUST   Many substances are being discovered as major causes of allergy that were never before suspected. Bits of dust from insect wings and other bug parts are one of these newly discovered causes. Just as ragweed, grass, and other pollens get into the air, so do the tiny disintegrated bits of debris that are associated with insects. Allergy can be produced by mayflies, silk cocoons, grasshoppers, ant eggs, houseflies, mosquitoes, bees, water fleas, mites, and fruit flies. With hundreds of millions of insects present in the air and in the ground, nearly all dust contains insect substances. You don't even have to be in direct contact with insects, just with ordinary dust.

The fact that insect dust can cause hayfever allergy may be the reason so many hayfever sufferers have not been helped by injections against ragweed and other common causes of allergies. For example, at Northwestern University Medical School, where much of the early work on insect dust was done, one woman came in who had had a stuffed-up nose and watery eyes for nearly all of her adult life. She had some symptoms the entire year and was severely disabled from May through October. Extensive testing to find the cause of her allergy failed. She was given drugs, but they did not give much relief. Allergists at Northwestern noticed several patients whose skin tests showed sensitivity to silk, but they were almost never exposed to silk fabrics. What caused the positive reaction? It turned out to be insects. So the allergists wondered whether that could be the problem patient's allergy. They prepared injections of insect extracts for her, and all of her symptoms disappeared in a few months.

Nearly 30 percent of all hayfever and asthma patients later tested were found to be sensitive to one or more insects. Now more and more different insects are being discovered as allergy-causers. Even cockroaches can be a cause. In fact, an estimated 10–15 million people in the United States are allergic to cockroaches, according to studies by epidemiologists at the National Institutes of Health and other allergists. Many hayfever and asthma patients have positive reactions to them.

The most troublesome insect is the house-dust mite (see the photo). The tiny (7,000 can fit on a fingernail) bodies of thousands of these mites and their waste products are frequently present in dust and are often really responsible for dust allergy.

House-dust mite hot spots include carpets, upholstered furniture, mattresses and pillows, and stuffed toys. They're there even if you

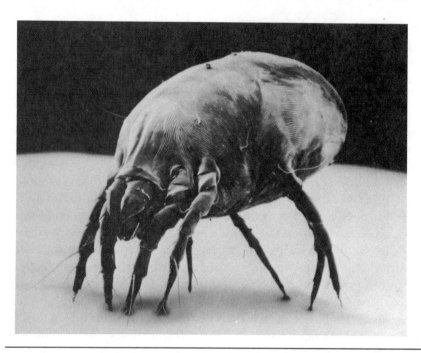

A house–dust mite. (*Source:* National Jewish Center for Immunology and Respiratory Medicine.)

are a very good housekeeper. A University of South Florida study found 10,000 of the beasts in a gram of furniture dust.

There is a do–it–yourself test to determine whether your home has mites, by testing your vacuum cleaner dust. Some experts say that about 90 percent of homes tested have the mites. But it's easiest, if you have an allergy, to see an allergist to learn whether you are allergic to mites, and if so to proceed with treating your carpet and other areas. One product is Acarosan® (check with your pharmacist or an allergy specialist to obtain it), made by the Fisons Corporation of Rochester, New York. It is a benzyl benzoate-based treatment product that can be dusted or sprayed on carpet and furniture to eliminate the invisible invaders for approximately six months. Another product, called Allergy Control™ Solution, manufactured by Allergy Control Products in Ridgefield, Connecticut, contains tannic acid, which actually changes the chemical makeup of the mite and its waste products so that it no longer produces an allergic reaction. It also has been found to work against cat danders. Allergy Control Products also has special filters for vacuum cleaners and nonplastic covers for pillows and mattresses.

House-Dust Mites
"Research has demonstrated that exposure to house-dust mite allergens in early childhood is an important determinant of the subsequent development of asthma."   *National Institute of Allergy and Infectious Diseases.*   "Mite infestation may be found in clean as well as poorly maintained homes."   Hospital Practice.

OTHER STEPS TO TAKE

- Eliminate dust-catchers. Store seldom-used things in plastic bags.
- Clean heating/air-conditioning filters frequently.
- For mites: wash all bedding in hot (at least 130°F) water every seven to ten days.
- For cockroaches: discourage cockroach populations by keeping your attic ventilated (cockroaches like to be where there is no air flow), use cockroach repellants, keep food off countertops, and take garbage out every evening rather than leaving it in the kitchen. Watch for a new product now under development— insulation that is impregnated with cockroach repellant.

Cockroaches: More of a Problem Than You Thought
"Allergy to cockroaches poses a significant threat to human health."   *U.S. Department of Agriculture.*   "About 61 percent of asthmatic persons are sensitive to cockroaches, and exposure can mean an asthma attack."   *Dr. Banan King, chief of allergy and clinical immunology at the University of Kentucky College of Medicine.*   "People simply cannot continue to view cockroaches as just a nasty nuisance."   *Dr. Richard Brenner, U.S. Department of Agriculture.*

Mold Allergy

Mold allergy, once thought to be rare, is now known to be a major cause of bronchial asthma, seasonal and perennial hayfever, and eczema.

Mold grows nearly everywhere. It spoils bread, rots fruit, mildews clothes. It grows in abundance on wheat, corn, oats, grasses, leaves, straw, hay, and even soil. Allergies to mold are frequently encountered among furniture repairers who work with old bedding and overstuffed furniture, among gardeners, farmers or botanists, and among others who work in damp or musty places.

In the house, molds are especially found in furniture and mattress dust and stuffed animal toys. Molds can grow in the shower, in humidifiers, air conditioners, and drip pans of refrigerators or their rubber door gaskets. An article in the *Journal of the American Medical Association* reports on a man who had allergic reactions to moldy water poured on the hot rocks in his sauna! Molds also attack paper products, wallpaper paste, paint, wood, cloth, and leather. They have been found on the underside of leaves of house plants, in foods, in damp cellars, and in summer cottages that have been closed for long periods. In damp areas be particularly careful of awnings, tents, draperies, window shades, wallpaper, canvas, and upholstered furniture and mattresses.

Even during winter, when the wind blows the soil dust, there are enough mold spores to produce symptoms in some sufferers. Suspect a mold allergy if your attacks occur in musty rooms, damp basements, barns, or similar places. If you smell something musty or moldy, then you've got it. People who react to mold usually have asthma or hayfever, with the same symptoms as those who are allergic to pollens, although eczema can also be caused. Many people are sensitive to both pollens and molds. All patients who have hayfever should be routinely tested with mold extracts also.

WHAT TO DO ABOUT MOLD ALLERGY

- As much as possible, all suspicious material such as old books, old furniture, and bedding should be removed from the environment.
- Damp cellars should be dried with dehumidifiers.
- Mold-proof paint should be used in place of wallpaper. Mold-inhibiting products can be sprayed or painted on walls and in cellars, but that must be repeated at regular intervals.

- In areas of high humidity take special care to see that shoes, gloves, suitcases, and clothing are not allowed to become mold-infested. Keep an electric light burning in a clothes closet to keep it warm and dry. For apartment dwellers, it's best to live above ground level, not in a basement.
- Allow adequate ventilation of rooms and storage areas.
- Clean mold-collecting places such as refrigerator drip pans frequently, and use a germicide. If you sneeze when the car air conditioner is on, have the tank capsule cleaned. (There may be mold in the air conditioner. In addition, it helps for the first few minutes to run the air conditioner with car windows open, since the mold usually is pushed out when the AC is first turned on.)
- Use glass shower doors, or if you have a shower curtain, wash it frequently.
- Use antimold tile cleaners in the bathroom shower area. You can use a commercial preparation or try a solution of household bleach and water. (If you dilute them, you can also use some mold retardants to prevent mold from growing on soil of house plants.)
- Don't overwater your plants; wet dirt encourages mold to form.

Your Pet May Be the Source of Your Problem

One of the biggest causes of allergies is dander from cats, dogs, and other animals. In fact, some allergists we interviewed called cats and dogs the single most important cause of allergies in children. The American Academy of Allergy and Immunology estimates that 20–30 percent of asthma patients may be allergic to animals, especially cats. Hayfever symptoms can be triggered by dander or by the dried saliva that comes to permeate the air from slobbering or fur licking, especially in cats. Some people get hives from a cat or dog's saliva.

Other animals can also cause allergy. Monkeys, guinea pigs, hamsters, rabbits, gerbils, and birds can all do it. Short hair, long hair, fuzz or feathers, it makes no difference. The smallest bird or chihuahua can cause an allergy. Even when the pet is kept in a box or cage in another room, the particles from their hairs or feathers can penetrate every corner of every room.

One child had been hospitalized four times with pneumonia before he was even one year old. Skin tests showed that he was sensitive to dog and cat hairs and to dust. The house was made as allergy-proof as possible, especially his bedroom, and the family dog and cat were given to friends who were caring people and loved animals. The boy's problems disappeared.

It may not even be a pet. One farmer discovered that he developed asthma whenever he went into the chicken coop attached to his house. One girl developed wheezing and sneezing whenever she fed pigeons in her backyard. And one woman's asthma was traced to sparrows nesting in vines under her bedroom window.

WHAT TO DO ABOUT ANIMAL ALLERGY If you or someone in your family has eczema, asthma, or a runny nose and you have an animal in the house, it should be the first thing you consider as a cause of the allergy. No matter how much you love your pet, you must consider parting with it. First, however, to make sure it is the cause, put your dog or cat in a kennel or with friends for several weeks. Clean the house thoroughly, vacuuming rugs, drapes, and furniture and washing down hard surfaces to get rid of all traces of dog hairs and dander. Continue vacuuming twice a week to remove lingering dander and hairs. If sniffing and sneezing stops or if the skin rash goes away, you can be almost sure it was the dog or cat that was causing the problem. However, if after this test you still have symptoms, then something other than your pet is causing the trouble. If the allergic person in your family has only a mild case of hayfever, it sometimes works to keep the pet outside and not allow it in the house. It also helps to wash your hands after playing with a dog or cat and to regularly wash the dog or cat. But if symptoms are severe, you need to get rid of the pet.

You May Be Allergic to a Food

You may have a reaction to any food. Those that people are most often allergic to are: shellfish, nuts, strawberries, milk, eggs, yeast, corn, and wheat. (However, sometimes a problem with milk can be a lactose intolerance rather than an allergy. The problem can often be managed by substituting lactose-reduced milk or by adding an enzyme called lactase to the milk. Several products, such as Lactaid® and Dairy-Eze®, are available at drug stores.)

You can also be allergic to food *additives,* such as synthetic colors, synthetic flavors, and preservatives. Common ones to watch for: yellow no. 5, BHA, BHT, benzoic acid, sulfites, and MSG.

Although there has been much controversy about it in the past, it appears that allergies can be a major influence in hyperactive children. *Pediatrics,* the journal of the American Academy of Pediatrics, has published a study by Dr. Bonnie Kaplan on hyperactive preschool boys. In the 10-week study, done in Canada, 24 hyperactive boys were given a diet that eliminated artificial colors and flavors, preservatives, chocolate, monosodium glutamate (MSG), and caffeine. The diet was low in simple sugars and also made free of dairy foods for children with a history of possible problems with cow's milk. More than half of the boys showed a reliable improvement in behavior. In addition, there often was improvement in bad breath, difficulty in falling asleep, and night awakenings. For more information on food and hyperactivity, write Feingold Associations of the U.S., P.O. Box 6550, Alexandria VA 22306.

Allergies and Behavior

"I think about all the mothers with children who don't know that bad behavior may be allergically induced...I used to think they were just nasty children and then I found that we can turn their nastiness on and off with food reactions."

Dr. Doris Rapp, pediatric allergist, Buffalo Environmental Allergy Center.

WHAT TO DO ABOUT FOOD ALLERGY If you think your symptoms are caused by a food, exclude the food from your diet for several weeks and see if your symptoms go away. Then after at least a month of being symptom-free, eat the food and see if you develop the symptoms again. (However, if your first reaction included hives or another general body reaction, you should see an allergist for testing. A second exposure could give you a more severe reaction.)

Watch out for other foods and even nonfood products related to your food troublemaker. If you are allergic to corn, for example, you should also avoid beer, corn-based gelatins, and many pastries, as well as starched shirts, bath powders, the glue on stamps and envelopes, chewing gum, and paper cups and plates. If you are allergic to eggs, you need to avoid pastries baked with egg, ice cream, sherbets, and many sauces.

Sulfites

The Food and Drug Administration banned the use of sulfites on raw fruits and vegetables in restaurant salad bars in 1986 because that was the main source of allergic reactions. But you can still find sulfites in most homes. If you are allergic to sulfites (sometimes asthmatic people have severe asthma attacks from them), watch for sulfites used as preservative in many breads, wines, raisins and other dried fruits, canned and frozen vegetables, and other foods. Read labels. Stick to fresh produce whenever possible. Look for products labeled "no preservatives added."

If your diet has to be restricted greatly because of your allergy, then you should work with a nutritionally oriented doctor to find a well-balanced diet that will give you all the proper vitamins and nutrients while keeping you away from the troublesome foods. Sometimes, if the allergy to a food is not severe, you can use a rotation diet worked out with your physician to eat the offending food no more than once a week.

If you have difficulty discovering a specific food that is causing your trouble, suspect a food additive. Do your best to buy only fresh, unprocessed foods that have no additives or preservatives. (For a list of organic food mail-order suppliers, send a long, self-addressed envelope and 50 cents in stamps to: Center for Science in the Public Interest (CSPI), 1501 16th Street NW, Washington DC 20036.)

The Case of the "Stupid Kid"

An eight-year-old boy had a behavior problem, was inattentive, and had poor grades. His teachers said he was stupid. An alert pediatrician found he had a hearing loss caused by an allergy. Influenced by ads for a chocolate syrup on TV, he had begun to drink a quart of chocolate milk a day. Two days after chocolate was eliminated from his diet, he began to improve.

You May Be Allergic to a Medicine

You may be allergic to the medicine itself, or, as in foods, you may be allergic to an additive. Penicillin, streptomycin, and sulfa drugs frequently produce allergic reactions, and a huge number of people are allergic to aspirin and related substances. One of the early astronauts had to drop out of the program because of aspirin sensitivity. Many people allergic to shellfish are also allergic to iodine in medicines.

Other medicines cause no trouble until the person goes into the sunlight, and then they have a photosensitivity reaction; among other symptoms, the skin may become red, swollen, blistered or scaly, or there may be dark blotches that last for years. Drugs that can cause sun-sensitivity reactions include sulfonamides, coal tar, and several antibiotic and antifungal agents and thiazides. Celery, lime juice, cyclamate and saccharin can cause sun sensitivity also.

You can even be allergic to the medicine you take for an allergy!

WHAT TO DO ABOUT ALLERGY TO MEDICINE

- When a medicine is prescribed for you, always ask what side effects might occur and what you should do if they do occur. Always tell the doctor about any other prescriptions or over-the-counter preparations you are taking, even hormones, vitamins, or herbs, since substances can sometimes react with each other.

- If at any time while you are taking a medicine you have any kind of side effect, immediately call your physician so that he or she can consider an alternative brand or different medicine. Do *not* stop taking the medicine on your own.

- Any time that a drug is prescribed to you, be sure to tell the prescribing doctor of any allergies you have had in the past, even mild reactions.

- If you think you are allergic to a medicine or an ingredient that sometimes appears in medicines, always read the labels of any medicine before you take it. If you are allergic to aspirin, for example, you will probably be allergic to any salicylate. You would need to be wary of such things as Alka-Seltzer®, Anacin®, APC®, Bufferin®, Darvon®, Excedrin®, Pepto-Bismol®, salicylate flavoring, some candy, chewing gum, soft drinks and gelatins, even green soap.

You May Be Allergic to Things You Touch

Contact dermatitis is a rash of the skin caused by something that you have touched, something that your skin has been in direct contact with. The skin itches or becomes red, often swells, or may have little bumps or blisters. The blisters may break and form crusts and scales.

Determining the cause of a contact dermatitis can be one of the most intriguing detective games in the whole field of allergy diagnosis and treatment. For example, if the folds of your skin don't have the rash, then a solid object is suspected. Fluid or semifluid materials tend to gather in folds and creases.

Contact dermatitis can be caused by a seemingly insignificant part of your life: many office workers with skin and eye irritations were found allergic to the chemicals in no-carbon copies. Dr. Tom Enta reported in *Canadian Family Physician* of a new diagnosis: blue-jean nickel button dermatitis. He found it occurring in women as a result of jeans that had a central fly with metallic snap buttons. People can be allergic to gold too.

The following are typical causes of allergic skin reactions.

NICKEL People with nickel allergy can get a skin rash from handling coins, as well as from wearing jewelry or wrist watches containing nickel alloys. Doctors, for example, report women coming in with what appears to be an infection of the earlobe, but which was caused by an allergy to the nickel in pierced earring posts.

RUBBER Rubber products frequently cause allergic contact dermatitis. It's not so much the rubber causing the trouble as the chemicals that have been added in manufacturing. Rubber products can be found in many places: rubber padding in dress shields, rubber edges of eyelash curlers, rubber gloves, boots, and so on.

CHROMATE You can be exposed to chromate (a product of chromic acid) in leather, matches, paints, disinfectants, bleaches, and glues. It often occurs in leather dye and can cause dermatitis of the feet. Some matchheads contain chromates, and perspiring fingers that touch matches can become contaminated and then touch other parts of the body.

SYNTHETIC RESINS Synthetic resins are sometimes found in wash-and-wear, drip-dry clothes. You can sometimes detect them in new clothing by a "laboratory" odor. Synthetic resins are also used in plastic jewelry, watchbands, fungicides, tanning materials, rubber, glossy paper, cigarette packages, and some photography products.

The Office at Home

"Carbonless copy paper (CCP) can cause potentially life-threatening allergic reactions in sensitive individuals. Writing on the top sheet of CCP causes microcapsules containing colorless dye to burst on the underside and release chemicals that react with a color-developing substance on the bottom copy and that also can cause skin rash, shortness of breath, headache and fatigue."

Dr. Frank P. LaMarte, University of Iowa College of Medicine in the Journal of the American Medical Association.

WHAT TO DO TO REDUCE SKIN RASHES

- If you tend to get "housewife eczema," protect your hands with cotton-lined plastic or rubber gloves while working. (Unlined ones will cause sweating and irritate the hands even more.) For nonwet work, use light cotton gloves.

- Don't use more soap and detergents than necessary when you clean or launder. Use mild cleaners rather than strong ones. Take care to rinse thoroughly.

- If you are allergic to wool, do not use wool clothing or blankets. If you sometimes wear wool anyway, at least take special precautions around the wrists, ankles, and neck to prevent contact of wool with these areas. Don't get on the floor if you have wool rugs.

- Keep as cool as possible; excess perspiration may cause a flare-up of a rash or irritate the skin.

- Avoid pressure of garments over the rash, such as tight clothes, rings, and watchbands.

- For relief, applying ice or compresses of cool tap water may sometimes be soothing.

- If a baby reacts to commercial lotions, try simple cooking oils or shortenings.

YOUR SPOUSE'S OR YOUR COSMETICS   Allergy to cosmetics can affect both men and women and occurs much more often than generally realized. Many women have drying and cracking of their lips after using certain lipsticks, and both men and women can be allergic to perfumes. There can be contact dermatitis where the cosmetic touches the skin, or there can be hives or respiratory symptoms. Redness and itching of the eyelids may be due to mascara, eyeshadow, eyeliner, or adhesive on false eyelashes, or they can be due to soap, hair dye, or nail polish transferred by rubbing the eyes. Dermatitis of the scalp can be caused by shampoos, hair tonics, hair dyes, permanent wave solutions, or hairsprays.

More than one romance has taken a turn for the worse when the boyfriend developed swollen lips every time he kissed his girl. One man who sold women's shoes had to change his job because the perfumes that most of his customers wore gave him asthma. Sometimes even the fragrance in scented facial tissue, toilet paper, or soap can cause a reaction.

Babies, too, can be allergic to their mother's cosmetics. The baby may have a rash or hives from direct contact, or may have a cough or runny nose. If your baby develops such symptoms, think about what is new in his or her environment, and include your cosmetics on the list of possible troublemakers. Try going for several weeks without makeup or perfume when you are around your baby and not using hairspray, and see if it makes a difference.

You may have a reaction to a cosmetic after you have changed to a new type or when a new ingredient is added to your regular brand, or it may suddenly and unexplainedly appear with the continued use of the same cosmetic even after years of use.

Allergy to cosmetics is not always easy to recognize. One woman had a stuffy nose, then for two months had an inflamed throat and sinus trouble, then she had a burning tongue for several days. She thought she had a severe cold and sinusitis and took antihistamines, throat lozenges, and nasal sprays, and then was given antibiotics. Finally, a new indelible lipstick was incriminated. The woman was told to discontinue it and was free of all symptoms in four days.

Another woman had red puffy eyelids, and burning and itching of the neck, under the arms, and on the abdomen. It seemed to be an allergic reaction, but her doctor could not figure out what caused it until she mentioned that her symptoms were most severe the day after her weekly visit to the beauty shop for a shampoo and manicure. Patch tests for the shampoo were negative, but the nail polish provided a strong reaction. The symptoms on the neck, arms, and abdomen appeared because she tended to rub her eyes and fiddle with her necklace and scratch her abdomen when reading in bed at night.

Two of the major offenders in cosmetics are orris root and karaya gum. They are often found in face powder, shaving cream, facial cream, sunburn lotion, shampoo, rouge, perfume, lipstick, soap, hair tonic, and also in items such as sachets, teething rings, toothpaste, dental adhesive powders, and some drugs and even foods such as certain brands of gelatin, ices, ice cream, salad dressings, pies, and gumdrops.

If you believe you have symptoms caused by cosmetics, then be particularly careful of orris root and karaya gum in all products. You can be careful to read labels, or buy only hypoallergenic brands of cosmetics, which have no indelible dyes, perfumes, or other substances that so often cause allergic reactions in the sensitive individual. One manufacturer of hypoallergenic cosmetics says their company has eliminated more than sixty ingredients that are ordinarily contained in cosmetics.

Experiment with different brands. You may often have a reaction to one brand of something but not to another.

PLANTS IN YOUR HOUSE Many plants besides poison ivy, poison oak, and poison sumac can cause reactions. Known troublemakers are gaillardia, buttercup, primrose, mayapple, poinsettia, chrysanthemum, philodendron, daisy, and tulip. Even dried plants can cause dermatitis, as can handling tulip bulbs or orange peels.

Fishermen can get a rash from using lacquered fishing rods manufactured in Japan. Voodoo dolls imported from Haiti and drink stirring sticks made from cashew nuts may produce a rash, and so can the rind of a mango.

Rules for Allergy-Proofing Your Home

The best way to fight any allergy is to avoid whatever is causing your problem: Keep the troublemakers out of your environment. Complete elimination isn't usually possible, but even partial correction of allergy-promoting conditions will be helpful. Carry out as many of these instructions as possible even though some may be difficult, and you will likely find allergy symptoms substantially improved.

- Have as little overstuffed furniture as possible, especially old upholstered furniture. Usually the older the furniture, the more allergy it causes.

- Keep furnishings simple. Keep things that are necessary as dust-free as possible. Avoid things that are likely to collect dust such as drapes, venetian blinds, knickknacks, books.
- Avoid shag, chenille fabrics, kapok, animal hairs, feather pillows.
- All bedding, including blankets and spreads, in the allergic person's room should be washable and should be washed frequently.
- Use covers on pillows, mattresses, and box springs.
- Children should have only washable toys.
- If you have hot air registers, put several layers of cheesecloth across and under the register to help filter out the dust coming through with the hot air.
- When you clean, be sure to clean under and behind furniture, the tops of doors, window frames, sills, moldings, lights, and closet shelves. Use a damp cloth rather than a feather-duster, and a damp mop rather than a dust mop. Have a professional cleaning service if necessary. (The allergic person should be out of the room when it is being cleaned.)
- Vacuuming twice a week is usually recommended if people with allergies live in the house and should include not only the furniture and rugs, but also any drapes, pillows, mattresses, or box springs.
- Try products that inhibit dust formation on furniture, rugs, and drapes. You can rinse fabrics in them, spray them on furniture, rugs, or car upholstery. Some hayfever victims even sponge them on their pet animals. (But be careful, you may be allergic to these products also.)
- See that your house has no tobacco smoke or kerosene or oil burners, and try to keep the hayfever sufferer away from insect sprays.
- During hayfever season keep the doors and windows of the house (or at least the bedroom) closed as much as possible to keep out pollen and to prevent drafts, which can stir up pollen and dust.
- Use central air-conditioning during pollen season to decrease the amount of pollens. Replace filters frequently. Some patients don't have to examine the filters. They know the morning they wake up sneezing that it's time to change the filter! You may need to hire a professional company to clean out your air

ducts of pollen, mites, and mold, especially in older houses. Also use an air conditioner in the car to filter out pollens and dust. Use the "recirculate" adjustment rather than "fresh air." Do not keep the temperature very cold, however, because chilling can irritate the nose and bronchial tubes. Moderate cooling with temperature not more than ten to twelve degrees lower than outdoors is generally recommended.

Keep Cool, Not Cold

Setting an air conditioner at too low a temperature can aggravate allergy symptoms. Don't get under 70°F.

Things to Consider if You Are Remodeling or Building a Home

Following are some things to consider that could help avoid allergens in the future.

- If there is a heating choice, electric heat or hot water is preferable to forced-air heat. The heating unit should be located in a separate room with an outside entrance, so that combustion does not produce fumes in the house.
- Install central air-conditioning. Consider installing in the system one of the new air filters called HEPA (high-efficiency particulate-arresting) or other systems with electronic or media air filters that are powerful enough to filter out pollen, dust, and mold. Before investing in an expensive air cleaner, however, check with your doctor. (You may be allergic to something other than dust, spores, or pollen; an air cleaner prescribed by your doctor is usually tax-deductible.)
- For the bathroom, consider sheet vinyls since they can be damp mopped and have no cracks to collect dust or mold spores. The flexible silicone rubber mastics offer the most impregnable seal between wall and tub.
- The clothes dryer should be vented to the outdoors.
- Check on the availability of a new insulation impregnated with cockroach repellant to keep roaches away.

Quick Summary

Allergies are the great masqueraders. If you or anyone in your family has a runny nose, itchy eyes, a cough, sneezing, a rash, digestive problems, or even emotional upsets, they may be due to an allergy to something in your home. What you're allergic to may be something you breathe, something you eat, or something you touch. In fact, it can be something as unthought of as gas fumes, cat dander, insect dust, or cosmetics.

It may take serious detective work to find the offending substance or substances, but the only way you will find relief will be to find the hidden problem and remove it from your environment.

ADDITIONAL RESOURCES

Allergy Testing Association
4727 Wilshire Blvd #610
Los Angeles CA 90010
800-522-8877

An information association that provides brochures and a referral list of physicians who perform in vitro allergy testing.

American Academy of Allergy and Immunology
611 E Wells St
Milwaukee WI 53202
800-822-2762

A professional medical organization, representing allergists in the United States, Canada, and other countries, that provides physician referral and public educational materials.

American College of Allergy and Immunology
800 E Northwest Highway #1080
Palatine IL 60067
708-359-2800

A professional medical organization, representing allergists, that provides patient education materials on allergy and asthma.

American Academy of Otolaryngic Allergy
8455 Collesville Rd Ste 745
Silver Spring MD 20910
301-588-1800

A professional medical organization of physicians that specializes in allergies affecting the ear, nose, and throat.

Asthma and Allergy Foundation of America
1717 Massachusetts Ave NW #305
Washington DC 20036
202-265-0265

A lay, voluntary organization, formed to help persons with asthma, allergies, and other disorders of the immune system, that provides physician contacts and educational materials.

Mothers of Asthmatics
10875 Main St #210
Fairfax VA 22030
703-385-4403

A nonprofit organization to help parents of children with asthma and allergies. Information for parents, schools, physicians, communities.

National Institute of Allergy and Infectious Diseases
National Institutes of Health Bldg 31, #7A32
Bethesda MD 20892
301-496-5717

Conducts and supports research on allergic, immunologic, and infectious diseases. Provides scientific articles for professionals and pamphlets for the general public.

National Jewish Center for Immunology and
    Respiratory Medicine
400 Jackson St
Denver CO 80206
800-222-LUNG

Treatment and research center for allergic, respiratory, and immunologic diseases. Brochures and other public education.

CHAPTER 7

PESTICIDES AND LAWN CARE CHEMICALS

Long-Term Health Dangers

An advertisement for an insecticide that appeared in the *San Antonio Express-News,* with unintentional humor, proclaimed: "Kill Your Aunts." The typo brings a smile to most of us—the lucky ones who haven't experienced the misery certain chemicals can cause. For example, in Washington D.C. in 1991 eight-year-old Jared Arminger, his voice quivering, testified before Congress: "I am interested in lawn care chemicals because I get sick from them. I get real sick when I am around lawn care pesticides. I can't think. I get depressed. A lot of other stuff happens to me like I don't listen. My nose runs, I get swollen glands, and my ears hurt. When I am around pesticides, I do not eat and I get diarrhea."

Jared told the Senate's Environment Subcommittee on Toxic Substances that, because of exposure to pesticides and lawn chemicals, he can't go to school or even go outside and play on nice days. Jared, from Baltimore, Maryland, was one of several witnesses who described the misery that pesticides have brought into their lives. The subcommittee also heard testimony from a woman who, because of partial paralysis, headaches, and vision loss, had to give up her career as a concert pianist after being sprayed with pesticides. Also testifying was a Dallas man who claims his health was ruined by the interaction of the lawn-care chemical diazinon with Tagamet®, a prescription drug for ulcers he was taking. A college student testified who sometimes sleeps in her car to avoid adverse health effects when pesticides are sprayed near her home.

Twenty-four states have enacted laws that require notification of chemically sensitive people before pesticide spraying by public agencies can be carried out. To be notified, chemically sensitive persons must register with their appropriate state agency. Check with your state health department's pesticide or toxicology office to find out if it has such a program.

An important member of the Senate's Environment Subcommittee on Toxic Substances, U.S. Senator Joseph Lieberman, says: "Too many of us fail to recognize that the chemicals that kill weeds and bugs are also powerful enough to threaten the environment and human health."

Sometimes just recognizing the potential danger is not enough. In Anniston, Alabama, a family is suing a national exterminating company for spraying their home with a termiticide containing chlordane, a chemical proven to cause cancer in animals and that can persist in the environment for 20 to 30 years or more. John and Velma Jean Tidball specifically asked the company if its termite treatment included chlordane and were told that it didn't. But after family members developed various ailments, they investigated further and found that chlordane had been used. They have since moved out of their home and have been unable to sell it.

Chlordane May Still Pose a Risk

From 1948 when it came onto the market until 1988 when it was banned by the EPA, chlordane and three additional chemically related compounds—heptachlor, aldrin, and dieldrin—were used to kill termites and other insects in 30 million homes. By 1983 the EPA had prohibited nearly all uses of the four pesticides *except for termite control*. The four compounds, called chlorinated cyclodienes, were allowed for termite control until 1988 because the EPA had concluded that, when these termiticides were applied correctly, residents of treated homes would not be exposed to them. However, the EPA banned the four compounds in 1988 because new studies showed that most chemicals used for subterranean termite control *can be found at low levels in the air of even properly treated homes*. In fact, approximately 90 percent of the homes treated with cyclodienes had detectable residue levels in the air one year after treatment. Chlordane has also been found in the soil of treated areas 20 to 30 or more years after treatment.

Other trade names for chlordane are Gold Crest® Termide, Gold Crest® C-100, Gold Crest® C.I.O.-20, Chlor-kill™, Octachlor™, Synklor™, and Topiclore™.

THE HEALTH DANGERS OF CYCLODIENES Besides causing cancer in lab animals, studies have linked chlordane inhalation to cases of infants' developing leukemia, aplastic anemia, and neuroblastoma (a type of brain cancer). The health risk to residents of houses sprayed with these chemicals depends on the levels of cyclodienes in the air, the amount of time residents have been exposed to them, and the sensitivity of the individual. Although the EPA emphasizes that the danger to particular individuals is low, it does view cyclodienes as "probable human carcinogens" and also has concerns about the long-term damage those substances can do to the liver and nervous system. Since large numbers of people have been exposed to cyclodienes and since these effects may result from exposure at lower levels than those associated with misuse, "the risk is a real one for a small percentage of the population," according to the EPA.

SYMPTOMS TO LOOK FOR Exposure to high levels of cyclodienes for prolonged periods can produce headaches, dizziness, muscle twitching, weakness, tingling sensations, and nausea. However, these symptoms may also indicate a wide variety of illnesses unrelated to cyclodiene exposure. If you experience such symptoms, see your doctor and express your concern about cyclodienes.

WHAT TO DO If your house was treated for subterranean termites prior to 1988, it is likely that chlordane or one of the other cyclodienes was used. If you suspect that your house has been sprayed or fumigated with a cyclodiene pesticide, you may want to have your house tested. Making the decision to test your home is a difficult one because it can be an expensive step.

Ask yourself the following questions to help decide whether or not to have a test:

- Do family members consistently show symptoms, such as those listed above, that could be caused by exposure to pesticides? Have you checked with your physician to rule out other possible causes?

- Are there any obvious, major structural flaws such as large cracks in the foundation? Could the cracks lead out to soil that may have been treated with cyclodiene-containing pesticides to prevent the entry of termites? Does your basement consistently leak?

- Do some residents of your home, especially those who show symptoms, spend a great deal of their time in the basement? For example, do they occupy bedrooms located in the basement?
- Does your home have air ducts located in the concrete slab or in the crawl space? Such homes are particularly vulnerable to earlier misapplications of cyclodiene-containing pesticides.
- Are there "chemical" odors inside your home? Do these odors increase when the heating or cooling system is in operation?

A yes answer to any of these questions is a strong indicator of past chlordane misapplication.

If you do decide to have your home tested, the EPA recommends you choose a laboratory proficient in both indoor air sampling and pesticide analysis. Costs vary depending on the amount and type of testing; they can range from $50 to $500. To locate a good laboratory in your area, you can call the National Pesticide Telecommunication Network at 800-858-7378. Or contact your state health agency (see Directory A under Termiticides) for advice on reputable local laboratories. When you locate a laboratory, ask for references about the expertise of the laboratory and statements about its experience regarding cyclodiene sampling and analysis.

WHAT DO YOUR TEST RESULTS MEAN?   The National Academy of Sciences published guidelines for airborne levels of certain termiticides in 1982, setting a level of five micrograms per cubic meter of air for cyclodienes. Although this level should not be viewed as a critical cutoff point, if you have levels higher than five micrograms, you should take corrective action. The EPA states that "for homes with high airborne levels of cyclodiene residues resulting from misapplication, building modification may be worthwhile." Such modifications must be designed on a case-by-case basis. Some experts have suggested cleaning contaminated household items, especially carpets, carpet pads, or curtains that may have been treated in the past with cyclodiene-containing products. *We go further—if your indoor air has been tested for cyclodiene residues and found to contain five micrograms per cubic meter or more, ask for a further test of your carpets, carpet pads, and/or curtains. If these household items are contaminated, replace them.* For homes with high airborne levels of cyclodiene residues, the only option may be an expensive one—replacing or relocating air ducts, replacing furnaces or ventilation systems with air exchangers, and/or sealing crawl space soil with a layer of concrete.

Even if your home has cyclodiene levels less than five micrograms, you may still take the following less stringent actions:

- Increase the circulation of clean air in your house. Weather permitting, periodically open windows and doors, and use fans to mix the air. In crawl spaces, add exterior vents, and install a fan to constantly force crawl space air to the outside. Take the other steps listed in Chapter 4 on ventilation.

- Fill cracks in the basement and ground floors and walls, joints between floors and walls, and openings around pipes, drains, and sumps. Use grout, caulk, or other sealants. Periodically check these areas for signs of new cracks or broken seals, since houses settle over time.

- Install a system that supplies outside air to appliances like clothes dryers and furnaces that now draw air from inside the house. Appliances that use indoor air actually help draw chemical vapors from the soil into the house through walls, floors, and basement.

- Check the condition of ducts in your crawl space or basement. Use duct tape to seal openings.

Other Pesticides That May Pose a Risk

The word *pesticide* comes from the combination of -*cide,* which is derived from the Latin verb that means *to kill* (as in homicide), and *pestis* for *plague.* Simply put, a pesticide is a killer of plagues and plague carriers. Pesticides include insecticides, herbicides, fungicides, rodenticides, fumigants, disinfectants, plant growth regulators, and other substances intended to kill or control unwanted insects, plants, fungi, mites, rodents, bacteria, or plants.

These chemical killers have been a boon to humanity. Until relatively recently in human history, people had to tolerate lice in their clothing, worms in their food, fleas in their bedding, and rodents in their homes and barns. Throughout history pests such as insects and rodents have carried diseases that have led to deadly epidemics. Famines resulted when locusts, fungi, and other pests destroyed crops.

After World War II, when many new chemicals were manufactured for military purposes, effective pesticide chemicals were developed and were viewed as wonder chemicals, examples of modern-day scientific miracles. Today, pesticides are being used with increasing and alarming frequency. Approximately 25,000 pesticide products are registered with the EPA for marketing and use in the United States. Total U.S. annual use of herbicide, insecticides, and fungicides is estimated at 1.1 billion pounds. *Time* Magazine (June 3, 1991) estimated that about 40 percent of the nation's private lawns are treated with pesticides. Runoff from these yards may threaten the safety of urban groundwater supplies and endanger health of neighbors.

It should therefore come as no surprise that environmentalists are now taking aim at such widespread pesticide use. Environmental concern first surfaced in the the 1960s, particularly after the publication of Rachel Carson's book, *Silent Spring*. People began to realize that pesticides not only can poison insects, plants, and animals, but also can poison people when used carelessly or inappropriately.

It took years for scientific data to accumulate, but accumulate it did. For instance, in 1986 the National Cancer Institute reported that Kansas farmers who were exposed to the chemical 2,4,-D—a popular herbicide used in both agriculture and home lawn care products—were more likely to develop non–Hodgkins disease lymphoma, a type of cancer, than those who were not exposed. A 1991 study revealed that dogs whose owners used a herbicide containing 2,4,-D are twice as likely to develop lymphatic cancer, a finding that suggests the plant-killing chemical may also pose a health risk to humans. A University of California study found that children whose parents use pesticides in the home had a seven times greater chance of developing childhood leukemia than those in pesticide–free homes. Other studies found that some early pesticides, such as DDT and other chlorinated hydrocarbon compounds that cause adverse health effects, persist almost indefinitely in the environment, moving up through the food chain from plants to birds, to fish, to mammals, and eventually to humans. As a result, DDT was banned in 1971. Most other chlorinated hydrocarbons have been banned or sharply restricted.

Meanwhile, scientists discovered that insects and other pests develop resistance or immunity to pesticides. In fact, according to the World Resources Institute, the number of species of insect pests resistant to one or more pesticides almost doubled between 1969 and 1980, costing U.S. farmers $150 million in crop losses. Since pests are becoming more resistant to pesticides, farmers have resorted to using more of these chemicals. And homeowners use three to six times as much pesticide per acre as farmers do!

This increase in pesticide use has led to increased consumer concern. According to the National Coalition Against the Misuse of Pesticides (NCAMP), 9 pesticides commonly used in lawn care may cause cancer, 10 may cause birth defects, 3 can affect reproduction, 9 can damage the liver or kidneys, 20 attack the nervous system, and 29 cause rashes or skin disease.

Consumers are so concerned about the health dangers of pesticides that they are increasingly calling the EPA-funded National Pesticide Telecommunications Hotline at 800-858-PEST. Operators working out of the Texas Technical University School of Medicine answer queries from consumers about specific pesticides. If the call is about a pesticide-related medical emergency, the call is immediately transferred to the Poison Control Center in New Mexico so that the caller can get prompt medical advice.

Five Home Pesticides That Concern Americans the Most

Hotline officials have tabulated their calls to find out which pesticides consumers are most concerned about. According to EPA health statistician Jerry Blondell, here are the top five pesticides of concern based on the number of calls to the Hotline during a recent four-year period (the second number listed is the number of people who expressed concern about potential or actual side effects including headache, nausea, increased sweating, muscle weakness, and fatigue):

- Chlorpyrifos, also known as Dursban®. The Hotline received about 15,401 calls for information as to dosage and toxicity. Of these calls, 1,470 involved people concerned about some type of potential adverse health effect caused by extensive exposure. Chlorpyrifos is found in pesticide products such as Black Flag® Roach and Ant Liquid Killer, Raid® Liquid Roach and Ant Killer Formula 1, and Hot Shot® Roach and Ant Killer as well as hundreds of other products.

- Diazinon. The Hotline received 7,704 calls about dosage and toxicity and 968 of those calls involved concern about some type of adverse health effect in humans. Diazinon is used as a pesticide to prevent bugs from infesting lawns and gardens. It's found in popular products such as Spectracide® Lawn and Garden Insect

Control, Ortho™ Diazinon Granules, Purina® Diazinon Insecticide 25E, and American Brand® Diazinon 4E, as well as hundreds of other pesticides.

- Malathion. The Hotline received 3,667 calls, with 541 individuals reporting adverse health effects. Malathion is found in many popular products including Ford's® 50 Percent Malathion Emulsifiable Liquid, Purina® Malathion Spray 54%, Security® Malathion MultiPurpose Spray, and Ferti-lome® Malathion Lawn and Garden Insect Control, as well as hundreds of other pesticide products.

- Carbarly, also known as Sevin. The Hotline received 2,562 calls, with 298 persons expressing concern about potential or actual adverse health effects. Carbarly is sold in many products including Security® Brand Sevin Spray, Sevin® Big 10 Dust, and Sevin® 5% Garden Dust; Ferti-lome® Bug Bait; Rigo® Garden Dust Special; and Pennington Liquid Sevin Insect Spray®; as well as hundreds of other pesticides.

- Pyrethrins. The Hotline received 3,190 calls, with 295 individuals reporting health adverse health effects. Pyrethrins are found in popular pesticide products such as Bengal® Flying Insect Killer, Raid House & Garden Spray®, and Blue Lustre® Flea Killer For Carpets, as well as hundreds of other pesticide products including personal bug repellents such as Deep Woods OFF!®.

Personal Bug Repellents May Cause Adverse Health Effects

Every summer we douse ourselves with chemical bug repellents to keep mosquitoes, ticks, and other insects from biting or stinging us.

What we don't realize is that these chemicals may have adverse health effects. Diethyltoluamide (DEET), an insect repellent developed for U.S. troops in Vietnam, is the main ingredient in many commercial mosquito sprays. However, in 1991 the EPA issued a consumer warning in response to several reports of DEET, in 100 percent solution, being used on children. Over the past decade, 10 individuals, most of them children, experienced adverse health reactions including headaches, convulsions, and unconsciousness. Although over 100 million people have used DEET safely, the EPA now advises people to avoid 100 percent solutions of DEET, never to use the substance over irritated or cut skin, to keep it away from the eyes and mouth, and to wash exposed skin with soap and water after returning indoors. Products that use Deet include Deep Woods OFF!®, Cutter® Insect Repellent, and Ticks OFF®.

With increasing awareness of tick-transmitted Lyme disease, many people are buying commercial tick repellents. Those most effective against ticks contain pyrethroids, synthetic derivatives of the pyrethrum plant. Natural pyrethrin dusts are among the safest tick powders for pets, says the Centers for Disease Control; however, synthetic pyrethroids, found in many pesticides, can cause severe allergic reactions in humans, according to EPA pesticide experts.

As an alternative to insecticides, many consumers are turning to Skin-So-Soft®, a bath oil with a nationwide reputation as a bug repellent. A recent consumer survey by New York's Mediamark Research company showed the Avon product to be the choice of one-fourth of all households that used repellents. This trend concerns some scientists who worry that none of the ingredients in Skin-So-Soft have been tested for full-strength use directly on people's skins. It should be noted that Avon markets the product as a perfumed bath oil, *not* as a bug repellent.

In response to concern about synthetic-chemical bug repellers, many people are turning to natural, herbal formulas. However, few of these herbal remedies have been safety tested by government agencies to determine if full-strength use directly on people's skins is safe. Still, herbal insect repellents have been around since ancient times. Citronella has been used for generations to repel mosquitoes; fresh peppermint and mountain mint, a common wild plant, are both effective in fending off ticks. Pennyroyal oil has also been used for years as a tick repellent; however, experts warn that pennyroyal should *not* be used during pregnancy because it might harm the fetus.

Many firms market herbal preparations using these insect-repelling ingredients but, because of government regulations, cannot advertise their products as bug repellents. Instead they label their products using a phrase like "herbal compound for outdoor use." Among those which have attracted wide followings:

- Green Ban™ for People and Green Ban™ Double Strength from Come To Your Senses, 321 Cedar Ave South, Minneapolis MN 55454; or call 612-399-0050. (Pregnant women should note that this product contains pennyroyal.)

- No Common Scents™ Herbal Insect Repellent from Lion & Lamb, 29-28 41st Ave, Long Island City NY 11101; or call 800-252-6288.
- Skeeter Shooo™ from EcoSafe Products, P.O. Box 1177, St. Augustine FL 32085; or call 800-274-7387.

Whenever using any type of bug repellent, first test it for several hours by using a small amount on a small portion of your skin. If you don't have any adverse reactions, it may be safe to try it over larger skin areas, but always be alert to the possibility of skin rashes or other adverse reactions.

OTHER SAFE WAYS TO KEEP BUGS AWAY According to anecdotal evidence, another safe way to keep bugs away is to take 100 mg. of vitamin B_1 before you go outdoors. The odor produced by the B_1 apparently drives bugs away. Eating cream of tartar tablets is also supposed to cause an odor on the skin that repels bugs.

To prevent bugs from being attracted to you, avoid brightly patterned or dark clothes. Instead wear white, tan, or light green. Avoid scented hairspray, cologne, or after-shave lotion. On picnics, avoid being around uncovered food for long periods of time. It attracts ants and other insects.

Avoid being around garbage areas, especially where fruit or open soda pop bottles or cans have been disposed. The sugar attracts bees, wasps, and hornets. Keep food or garbage covered or tightly wrapped.

FOOD SAFETY Consumers are also concerned about their food being safe from pesticide contamination. Although some experts fear that, without pesticides, American agricultural production would drop by at least 25 percent, environmentalists point to studies showing that farmers who use crop rotation and no chemicals actually get higher yields.

Under the Federal Insecticide, Fungicide, and Rodenticide Act, the EPA currently registers and regulates more than 25,000 pesticide products derived from about 600 basic chemical products. The EPA's task is to ensure that the risks pesticides pose to human health and the environment do not outweigh the many benefits that pesticides provide. You can help by making informed decisions about pesticide use in and around your home.

Keeping Insects and Other Pests Away from Your Home

PREVENT PEST INVASIONS IN THE FIRST PLACE   The first and most important step in pest control is to attempt to prevent the pest population from invading your home in the first place. Experts at the National Pest Control Association advise:

- Store garbage containers in dry, bright locations.
- Inspect plants for pests before bringing them indoors.
- Keep cupboards clean, and store sugar, flour, rice, and other nonrefrigerated foods in airtight containers or in the refrigerator.
- Seal or caulk any openings around windows, doorframes, or pipes through which pests can enter. Every time you fill in a crack with caulk, you reduce the number of roaches that may make your home *their* home. Roaches tend to reproduce in the security of a very small space, as narrow as $\frac{1}{64}$ of an inch, so fill even small cracks. And you can stuff steel wool around openings for pipes, which will also keep mice out.
- Prevent termite infestation by making sure wooden building materials do not come into direct contact with the soil. Treat wood posts and trellises with wood preservative to discourage termites.
- Store firewood, scrap wood, and other sources of cellulose away from the home.
- Make sure the soil around and under your home is well drained and that crawl spaces are dry and well ventilated.
- Make an annual inspection of your home, probing wood near the foundation with screwdriver or ice pick. Soft spots, holes in the wood, or missing chunks may be signs of termites at work. Periodic inspections ensure that you'll catch termites in the early stages when localized pest control treatments can control them.

ALTERNATIVE NONCHEMICAL METHODS OF PEST CONTROL   One California pest control firm uses liquid nitrogen to freeze termites. The Tallon Termite & Pest Control Co. of Long Beach, California, is a pioneer in killing termites by pouring liquid nitrogen, at $-20°$, into walls and other infested areas. The company also uses a heat treatment that heats localized areas to as much as 200° to kill the pests. Since wood doesn't burn until the temperature reaches 400°F, there is a wide margin of safety. Check with pest control companies in your area to see if such methods are available. Even though you may not have access to such innovative pest control methods, depending on the pest, there may be alternatives to chemical pesticides. For instance, if you have a gypsy moth problem, some exterminators use a biological pesticide — *Bacillus thuringiensis* — to rid your home of these pests.

Bacillus thuringiensis is an example of a naturally occurring microorganism that is used to control pests. Such microorganisms were first registered as pesticides in the late 1940s. Today there are 14 naturally occurring "good guy" bacteria, fungi, viruses, and protozoans that are registered in about 100 products used in home and garden applications, as well as in agriculture, forestry, and mosquito control. These products are pest-specific and are of low toxicity to humans. Ask your pest control company or county extension agent about such products. (The county extension agents and staff are representatives of the land grant university in your state and the U.S. Department of Agriculture's Federal Extension Service. In many instances, their offices are listed in the phonebook under *county*. Sometimes they can be found listed under *U.S. government* or *state government* because extension agencies are partially funded by the USDA Extension Service, your state, and your county government.)

Also check with local garden centers and mail-order garden catalogs for nonpolluting pesticides and fertilizers. For example, a product called Nemout® contains a nonharmful fungus that destroys nematodes, and a product called Flourish Grow Mor supplies potassium directly to plant foliage in small amounts rather than drenching the soil.

There are nontoxic roach and rodent killers you can make yourself. Here's how to make them.

Recipe for a Nontoxic Roach Killer

8 ozs. of baking soda
1/2 cup flour
1/8 cup sugar
1/2 chopped small onion
1/4 cup shortening or bacon drippings

Mix the shortening or bacon drippings with the sugar. Mix baking soda, flour, and onion; then add to shortening mixture. Blend well. Add enough water to form a soft dough. Shape into small balls. Place these balls in open plastic sandwich bags around the house in areas prone to roaches.

The baking soda gives off carbon dioxide gas in reaction with the roach's stomach acids. Since roaches are unable to belch, this kills them. Warning: Keep out of reach of children and pets, as large amounts can be toxic.

Nontoxic mouse repellent. Mice can't stand peppermint. Make a very strong peppermint tea, and after it cools, strain it and pour into a spray bottle. Spray where mice are likely to go. Repeat regularly.

Killing ants. Put a tablespoon of household laundry or dish detergent in a plastic spray pump bottle and fill it with water. Shake well. A squirt of sudsy water will kill ants when they appear.

If You Must Use Chemical Pesticides, Do It Safely

An EPA nationwide survey of household pesticide use indicated that 9 out of 10 American households use pesticides; but less than 50 percent of the people in the survey read pesticide labels for information regarding application procedures and preventive measures, and only 9 percent used pesticides with caution.

Why are people so blasé about pesticides? A chief reason is that in our modern society most people are in a hurry. They are used to reaching for a product that promises a quick fix to whatever pest problem they have. By not taking time to read labels, they don't recognize that the product can be dangerous. Remember, just as "pests" can be anything from cockroaches in your kitchen to algae in your swimming pool, pesticides include insecticides, herbicides, fungicides, rodenticides, disinfectants, and plant growth regulators—anything that kills or otherwise controls a pest of any kind. Take care with these products.

If you decide that chemical treatment is the best solution to your problem, then you need to decide whether to hire a professional pest control company or try to control the pests yourself.

If you decide to do it yourself, before you decide which product to use, you need to identify the pest and then find out what products are recommended for control of that pest. Ask experts or read labels to learn about the products' active ingredients, the ones that kill or otherwise neutralize the pest. A label will list active ingredients, the target pests, and the sites where the product may be used, for instance, indoors, on lawns, or in swimming pools. Be sure the site of your pest problem is listed. If it isn't, *do not* use the product.

Other questions to ask: Is it a "broad-spectrum" product (effective against a broad range of pests) or is it "selective" (effective against only a few pest species)? Which is best for your particular needs? If you have a roach problem, you may want to purchase a specific product designed to kill roaches. If you have a problem with an unidentified bug eating your flowers, you may need a broad-spectrum product. Either way, find out how rapidly the active ingredient in the product breaks down once it is introduced into the environment. Has it ever been suspected of causing adverse health effects? Chlordane, for example, was used for years after it was suspected of causing health problems. You might not want to take the risk with a product that even experts cannot verify as safe.

Other questions worth considering include: Is the product toxic to nontarget wildlife and to house pets? Is it known, or suspected, to leach through the soil into groundwater?

Besides the label, sources of information include the store where you purchased the pesticide, your County Extension Service, the experts of your state listed in Directory A, your state pesticide agency, or your regional EPA office.

When you have your facts together, you should choose the least toxic pesticide that can achieve the results. Then choose the formulation (and thus the method of application) that best suits your site and the pest you are seeking to control. The most common types of home-use pesticide formulations include:

- Solutions, containing the active ingredient and one or more additives, which readily mix with water

- Aerosols, which contain one or more active ingredients and a solvent

- Dusts, which contain active ingredients plus a very fine, dry, inert carrier such as clay, talc, or volcanic ash (dusts are applied dry)

- Granulars, which are similar to dusts, but with larger and heavier particles that settle and stay on the floor, in cracks, and in floor boards

- Baits, in which the active ingredients are mixed with food or other substances to attract the pest (not recommended if you have small children or pets in the home)
- Wetable powders, which are dry, finely ground formulations that are generally mixed with water for spray application

Whatever the type of formulation chosen, prepare only the amount you need for each application. Be careful not to inadvertently spray or otherwise contaminate yourself or others.

Application technique and timing of the application are every bit as important as the pesticide used. Again, read the label for specific instructions. We've said "read the label" several times, but it's important advice that deserves to be repeated. Read the label before you buy a product, before you mix it, before you apply it, before you store it, and before you throw it away. The directions are there for a good purpose: to help you achieve maximum benefits with minimum risk. (Notice we didn't say "maximum benefits with safety." Even the "safest" pesticide carries some minimum risk. It's up to you as a concerned consumer to become knowledgeable and to assume the level of risk you feel comfortable with.)

DETERMINING CORRECT DOSAGE There is usually no room on pesticide labels to include illustrative examples showing the multitude of home-use applications and how to dilute these products. The labels may inadvertently encourage preparation of more pesticide than is needed. Since the excess could contribute to overuse, safety problems related to storage and disposal, or simply the wastage of unused pesticide, the EPA, in its booklet *Citizen's Guide to Pesticides*, gives the following advice for determining the minimum quantity of pesticide needed for a particular situation.

> For example, the product label says, "For the control of aphids on tomatoes mix 8 fluid ounces of pesticide into 1 gallon water and spray until foliage is wet." Your experience has been that your 6 tomato plants require only 1 quart of pesticide to wet all the foliage. Therefore, only 2 fluid ounces of the pesticide should be mixed into 1 quart of water. Why? Because a quart is one-fourth of a gallon, and 2 fluid ounces mixed into 1 quart makes the same strength spray recommended by the label, but in a quantity that can be used up all at once.

Consumers can solve problems similar to this one with careful arithmetic, good measurements, and intelligent use of the Common Equivalents Charts that follow this section.

How to measure. If you need to determine the size of a square or rectangular area, such as a lawn for herbicide application, measure and multiply the length times the width. For example, an area 10 feet long by 8 feet wide contains 80 square feet (sq. ft.). Or area measurements may involve square yards (1 square yard equals 9 sq. ft.).

If you need to determine the volume of a space such as a room, first measure it and then multiply the room's length, width, and height. For example, a space 10 feet long, 8 feet wide, and 8 feet high contains a volume of 640 cubic feet (cu. ft.). You would use this procedure, for instance, for the release of an aerosol pesticide to control cockroaches.

Most *residential use* pesticides are measured in terms of volume. Some common equivalents are:

1 gallon equals 128 fluid ounces (fl. oz.)
1 gallon also equals 4 quarts (qt.)
1 gallon also equals 8 pints (pt.)
1 gallon also equals 16 cups
1 quart equals 32 fl. oz.
1 quart equals 2 pt.
1 quart equals 4 cups
1 pint equals 16 fl. oz.
1 pint equals 2 cups
1 cup equals 8 fl. oz.
1 tablespoon (tbsp.) equals 1/2 fl. oz. or 3 teaspoons (tsp.)
1 teaspoon equals 1/6 fl. oz.

The *Common Equivalents Chart* on page 113 provides examples to help you convert label information to your specific use situations. "Amount" can be any "unit" of pesticide quantity.

HOW TO DECIPHER PESTICIDE LABELS

- Check the label to make sure the pesticide product bears an EPA registration number. All pesticides legally marketed must bear an EPA-approved label that tells how dangerous they are. Look for one of the warning signal words on the label to tell you how poisonous a pesticide is if swallowed, inhaled, or absorbed through the skin.

Common Equivalents Chart

Pesticide Label Says Mix Amount of Pesticide	Equivalents 1 qt. water	1 pt. water
8 units per 1 gal. water	2 units	1 unit
16 units per 1 gal. water	4 units	2 units
32 units per 1 gal. water	8 units	4 units

Pesticide Label Says Apply Amount of Pesticide	Equivalents 20,000 sq. ft.	10,000 sq. ft.	500 sq. ft.
1 unit per 1,000 sq. ft.	20 units	10 units	$\frac{1}{2}$ unit
2 units per 1,000 sq. ft.	40 units	20 units	1 unit
5 units per 1,000 sq. ft.	100 units	50 units	$2\frac{1}{2}$ units
10 units per 1,000 sq. ft.	200 units	100 units	5 units

Pesticide Label Says Release Aerosol Cans	Equivalents 20,000 cu. ft.	10,000 cu. ft.	5,000 cu. ft.
1 unit per 10,000 cu. ft.	2 cans	1 can	Don't use
1 unit per 5,000 cu. ft.	4 cans	2 cans	1 can
1 unit per 2,500 cu. ft.	8 cans	4 cans	2 cans

"DANGER" means highly poisonous.
"WARNING" means moderately poisonous.
"CAUTION" means least hazardous.

- The label will also warn about whether or not a pesticide is restricted for use only by state-certified pest control operators. Do not use a restricted-use pesticide unless you have special training to do so. Such pesticides are simply too dangerous for application by an untrained person.

TIPS FOR HANDLING PESTICIDES

- Before using a pesticide product, know what to do in case of accidental poisoning. Read the label; it tells what to do in the event of poisoning.
- Follow directions carefully. Use only the amount directed and under the conditions specified and only for the purpose listed. Don't arbitrarily increase the amount of pesticide. Increasing the amount does *not* kill more bugs and can be harmful to you or others.

- Wear whatever degree of protective clothing the label recommends: long sleeves or pants, impervious vinyl or rubber gloves (not canvas or leather ones), footwear, hat, safety goggles, and a respirator. Personal protective clothing is usually available at home building supply stores.

- If you must mix or dilute the pesticide, do so outdoors or in a well-ventilated area. Again, mix only the amount you need, and use the recommended proportions.

- Keep children and pets away from areas where you mix or apply pesticides. Remove toys from the area. Remove birds and pets; cover aquariums and fish bowls.

- If spillage occurs, clean it up promptly. Don't just wash it away. Instead, sprinkle with sawdust or kitty litter, and sweep it into a plastic garbage bag. Dispose at a hazardous waste facility if your community has one. If not, dispose of it with the rest of your trash.

- Remove food, dishes, pots, pans, and other utensils before treating kitchen cabinets. Cover countertops and shelves to avoid getting pesticides on the surfaces. To be doubly safe after any application of pesticide in the kitchen, clean counter tops and shelves with a damp paper towel.

- When applying pesticide outdoors, close the windows of your home. Cover fish ponds and birdbaths. Avoid applying pesticides near a well.

- Allow adequate ventilation when applying pesticides indoors. Go away from the treated areas for at least the length of time prescribed by the label.

- Never place rodent or insect baits where small children or pets can reach them.

- Avoid overapplication, especially when treating lawn, shrubs, or garden. Runoff or seepage from excess pesticides can contaminate water supplies. Excess spray may also leave harmful residues on home-grown produce.

- Keep herbicides away from nontarget plants.

- Avoid applying pesticide to blooming plants, especially if you see bees or other pollinating insects around them. Avoid birds' nests when spraying trees.

- Never use spray or dust pesticides outdoors on a windy day.

- Never transfer pesticides to containers not intended for them, such as empty soft drink bottles. Keep pesticides in containers clearly and prominently identified as to contents. Properly refasten all childproof caps.

- Do not smoke while applying pesticides. It's too easy to carry traces of the pesticides from hand to mouth. Also, some pesticide products are flammable.

- Avoid touching face or other bare skin with contaminated gloves or clothing.

- Wash hands and face before eating, drinking, toileting, using tobacco, or taking other breaks.

- After the job is done, to remove chemical residues, use a garden hose to triple rinse tools or equipment used to mix or apply the chemicals.

- Prerinse outdoors the clothing that you wore when applying the pesticide. To prevent tracking chemicals inside, also rinse boots and shoes. Wash the clothes separately from the family laundry, in a heavy-duty detergent. Wash at least twice. Dry outside to avoid pesticide residues in the dryer. Remember to thoroughly rinse your washer by running it empty through at least another entire washing cycle using detergent. If fabric clothing has been saturated with a concentrated, highly toxic pesticide, don't bother washing it. Throw it away. Place the clothing in a plastic trash bag, close it tightly and dispose of it, along with your empty pesticide containers, if at all possible at a hazardous waste disposal facility.

- Shower and shampoo thoroughly after the pesticide application job is done.

- Later, evaluate the results of your pesticide use. Are the results worth the risks and hassle involved in using chemical pesticides?

How to Choose a Pest Control Company

If you decide you need the services of a professional exterminator, here are questions you should ask before hiring one.

- Does the pest control company have a good track record? Don't rely on company salespeople to answer this question. Research the answer yourself; ask neighbors and friends. Have any of them dealt with the company before? Were they satisfied with the service they received? Call the Better Business Bureau or local consumer office to determine if they have received any valid complaints about the company.

- Does the company have insurance? What kind? Can the salesperson show some documentation to prove the company is insured? The pest control company should have liability insurance that includes insurance for sudden and accidental pollution and that gives the homeowner protection should an accident occur while pesticides are being applied.

- Is the company licensed? Most states have regulatory agencies that issue state pest control licenses. Although the qualifications for a license vary from state to state, the license usually presents minimum requirements designed to protect you and your family. One such minimum requirement is that there be a certified pesticide applicator present at *the company office* to supervise the work of exterminators using restricted-use pesticides. (Certified applicators are formally trained and "certified" as qualified to use or supervise the use of restricted pesticides.) Ask that a "certified applicator" actually apply or supervise the application of chemicals to your home. Again, note that most states only require that the "certified applicator" merely be in the company's office. What good can he or she do from there, when a less trained person is about to make a mistake and misapply chemicals?

- Is the company affiliated with a professional pest control association? Professional associations keep members informed of new developments in pest control methods, safety, training, research, and regulation. They also have codes of ethics that members agree to abide by.

- Does the company stand behind its work? What guarantees does the company make? Be sure to find out what you must do to keep your part of the bargain. For example, in the case of termite control treatments, a guarantee may be invalidated if structural alterations are made without prior notice to the pest control company.

- Is the company willing and able to discuss all the details of the treatment proposed for your home?

- Will the pest control company, after inspecting your premises, offer a detailed control program in writing? It should specify what pests are to be controlled, the extent of the current infestation, what degree of control is to be expected, and what pesticide formulation and application will be used. It should also specify what alternatives to the formulation and techniques could be used instead. The company should have in writing special instructions for reducing your exposure to the pesticide (such as vacating the house, emptying the cupboards, removing pets, and so on) and how to minimize your pest control problems in the future.

- Finally, since contracts are documents jointly developed, you should add any safety concerns such as allergies or the fact you have young children or your elderly parents in the home. Get assurances in writing that application of the chemicals will not cause ill effects in the children or the elderly.

Storing and Disposing Pesticides Safely

The following tips on home storage and disposal may help you avoid tragedy in your home.

STORAGE

- To reduce storage problems, buy only enough product to carry you through the use season, and mix only the amount you need for the job at hand.
- Store pesticides away from children and pets as soon as you bring them into the house and again immediately after each use. A locked cabinet in a well-ventilated utility area or garden shed is best.
- Store flammable pesticides outside living quarters and away from ignition sources.
- Never put pesticides in cabinets with, or near, food or medical supplies—or near heat. Always store pesticides in their original containers, complete with labels that list ingredients, directions for use, and antidotes in case of accidental poisoning. Apply transparent tape over the label to keep it legible. If you have any doubts about the contents of a pesticide container, throw it out. (See disposal advice that follows.) Never reuse empty pesticide containers. Empty pesticide containers can be as hazardous as full ones because of the residues remaining inside. It's unlikely, says

the EPA, that these residues can ever be completely removed; so never attempt to clean them for reuse.

- Is your home on a flood plain? Avoid storing pesticides in places where flooding is possible, or in open places where they might spill or leak into the environment.

DISPOSAL   Follow directions on the label concerning how to dispose of the product and its container. If directions are illegible, the EPA advises the following:

- To dispose of less than a full container of a liquid pesticide, leave it in its original container with the cap securely in place to prevent spills or leaks. Wrap the container in several layers of newspapers and tie securely.

- Call your municipal or county government to check whether your community has a hazardous waste disposal site or a special pickup for toxic substances. If not, the EPA says it's okay to place a small quantity of pesticides, wrapped in the manner described, in a covered trash can for routine collection with garbage. Treated in this manner, small quantities of pesticides are not hazardous to trash collectors or to the environment. (In a properly operated municipal, sanitary landfill, the pesticides will be sufficiently diluted to pose no hazardous effects to individuals or the environment.)

- If you do not have a regular trash collection service, bury empty pesticide containers at least 18 inches deep in a place on your property away from water sources, away from where you grow or may grow food in the future and away from where children may play.

- Never puncture a pressurized pesticide container. It could explode.

- Do not pour leftover pesticides down the sink or into the toilet. Chemicals in the pesticides could interfere with the operation of septic tanks and are likely to pollute waterways. (Many municipal wastewater treatment systems cannot remove all pesticide residues.)

Quick Summary

Chemical pesticides must be used very carefully to achieve results without harming you, your family, or the environment. Some points to consider before deciding to use pesticides include: (1) The results are generally only temporary; (2) They are often more expensive than preventive or other methods. Therefore, consider using preventive and nonchemical treatments instead of chemical ones or at least alternating nonchemical methods with them. This reduces the buildup of chemicals after repeated applications. Also, evaluate the results of your pesticide use, comparing before- and after-treatment conditions. Weigh the benefits of short-term chemical control against the benefits of long-term control using alternative methods.

ADDITIONAL RESOURCES

- *Termiticides, Consumer Information*, a pamphlet by the EPA published January 1988. Write: EPA, 401 M Street SW, Washington DC 20460.

- *A Consumer's Guide to Safer Pesticide Use*, by the EPA Office of Public Affairs. Write: EPA's Public Information Center, 401 M Street SW, Washington DC 20460. For specific tips on the safe use of pesticides, write to the same address for the free brochure *A Citizen's Guide to Pesticides*.

- *Common Sense Pest Control* is a quarterly that summarizes recent findings on how to control pests using environmentally sound methods. It and *IPM Practitioner*, a digest of the scientific literature on how to control pests using environmentally sound methods that is issued 10 times a year, are both available for $45 each from Bio-Integral Resource Center, P.O. Box 7414, Berkeley CA 94707.

- *Common Sense Pest Control: Least-Toxic Solutions for Your Home, Garden, Pets, and Community*, by William Olkowski, Ph.D., Sheila Daar, and Helga Olkowski is a 720-page book on how to control plant and insect pests. A main selection of The Garden Book Club, it was published June 1991 by Taunton Publications and costs $39.95.

- To have your home checked for pesticide residue, call your state health department (see Directory A). For further information on pesticides, call the EPA's toll-free Pesticide Hotline at 800-858-7378.

CHAPTER 8

RISKY WATERS

Is Your Water Safe?

When Jane Myers of Pittsfield, Massachusetts felt too sick to do her Christmas shopping, she thought her fatigue, muscle aches, and diarrhea were caused by the flu—until she discovered that practically everyone in her neighborhood felt the same. Eventually more than 700 Pittsfield residents were found to have giardiasis, caused by a parasite transmitted in water. Faulty filtration of the Pittsfield water supply was to blame.

Water is a vital resource, essential to life. More than half of all Americans use public water systems drawn from rivers, lakes, and open reservoirs; the rest get drinking water from wells and springs that come from groundwaters—water in underground saturated beds of sand and gravel. Most Americans take availability of safe drinking water for granted, yet from coast to coast our rivers, lakes, groundwaters, and other essential water sources are becoming polluted with industrial, agricultural, and municipal wastes. In the early part of summer, half of all rivers and streams in America's farm belt are laced with unhealthy levels of pesticides.

One Out of Six of Us May Be Drinking Contaminated Water
Various governmental agencies and environmental organizations have repeatedly reported that fully 42 million Americans, about one in every six, are drinking water contaminated at dangerously high levels.

Since 1974, more than 2,100 organic and inorganic contaminants have been identified nationwide in drinking water at various levels by numerous federal and state survey programs, according to Ralph Nader's Center for Study of Responsive Law. Of the 2,100 contaminants, 190 are known or suspected to cause adverse health effects (including cancer) at certain levels of concentration.

No matter where our water comes from, we should inquire as to its safety. Overwhelming scientific evidence has been mounting that new chemicals and microbiological contaminants have begun to seriously degrade the quality of both our surface water and our groundwater. Since 1980, reports warning about water pollution have been issued by such prestigious organizations as the American Chemical Society, Institute of Professional Geologists, National Academy of Science, Natural Resources Defense Council, American Petroleum Institute, and the Office of Technology Assessment, as well as the EPA.

Nearly two decades after Congress passed the Safe Drinking Water Act of 1974, the water flowing from our nation's taps is anything but pristine, according to *Consumer Reports* magazine. Not all experts agree, but the bottom line, according to many government and independent studies, is:

- One in six people drink water with excessive amounts of lead, the heavy metal that impairs the I.Q. of children.
- Waterborne radon may cause more cancer deaths than all other drinking-water contaminants combined.
- Bacteria in water may be responsible for one in three cases of gastrointestinal illness.

Are You Getting Sick Because of Contaminated Water?

Yet according to the Centers for Disease Control (CDC) there are only about 7,400 reported cases of drinking-water–related illness documented each year. Why the discrepancy between the estimates and reported cases? Although the relatively small annual number of reported cases — in a nation of over 250 million people — may at first seem reassuring, the CDC believes this figure is only a fraction of the total water-caused illnesses that actually occur. Some experts believe that the real number may be as much as 25 times higher.

SYMPTOMS AND ILLNESSES CAUSED BY CONTAMINATED WATER

Microorganisms are responsible for more reported cases of acute illness than any other water contaminants. "Many people get sick and experience symptoms such as diarrhea and suffer through the episodes without reporting it to anyone," says Anita Highsmith, chief of the Water Quality Laboratory of the Centers for Disease Control.

The following signs and symptoms can be caused by contaminated water: Bacteria, viruses, or parasites in water can cause flulike symptoms such as muscle aches, fatigue, and gastrointestinal upset including diarrhea, nausea, and vomiting with or without fever. Symptoms such as diarrhea can last for one to two days and then disappear or, if caused by parasitic contamination of the water, last for several weeks and require medical treatment. Microorganisms can also cause serious illnesses such as typhus, cholera, and hepatitis A, which are the most serious of several bacterial, protozoan, and viral diseases known to be transmitted to humans through water. Other bacterial diseases include dysentery, typhoid, and salmonellosis infections. Typhoid and a related typhoid disease, paratyphoid, are characterized by headache, body pain, high fever, and constipation alternating with diarrhea, whereas cholera, dysentery, and salmonellosis are all typified by severe diarrhea and vomiting.

"If people of all ages and sexes in the same geographic area get sick about the same time, as did those in Pittsfield, Massachusetts, it's a tip-off that the cause is some sort of water contamination," states Dr. Dennis Juranek, chief of epidemiology at the Centers for Disease Control.

Drinking water contaminants can be conveniently grouped into three other categories besides microbiological contamination:

Radionuclides, including radium-226 and -228, uranium, and radon, are of great concern as contaminants of drinking water because they can cause cancer. As many as 17 million people living in New Jersey, New England, and in western mountain states face the radon threat because that radioactive gas permeates groundwater in those regions.

Organic contaminants of drinking water include hydrocarbons, benzene, chlorobenzenes, pesticides, polychlorinated biphenyls, and chlorinated alkanes such as chloroform, trichloroethylene, tetrachloroethylene, carbon tetrachloride, methylene chloride, and vinyl chloride. Most of these are known or suspected cancer causers. They also can cause chronic skin irritations, itchy eyes, and respiratory problems.

Inorganic contaminants are arsenic, cadmium, chromium, cyanide, fluoride, lead, mercury, nitrates, and selenium. Both cyanide and arsenic are poisons at certain concentrations. Cadmium can cause kidney damage; high concentrations of chromium and selenium can cause cancer and too much fluoride can cause hardening of the bones. Lead and mercury play havoc with the human nervous systems.

Excessive concentrations of nitrate, generated by the breakdown of fertilizer and sewage, also can find its way into groundwater. Once ingested, nitrate can be transformed in the stomach and bladder into compounds called nitrosamines, potent carcinogens which have been found to cause cancer and mutations in rats. Research on the health effects in humans is shockingly sketchy. Nitrate can react with hemoglobin in the blood to cause an anemia named methemoglobinemia. The condition, also known as blue baby syndrome, can occur at any age, but occurs most frequently in infants 3 to 12 months old. Bacteria within the baby's stomach convert the nitrates to nitrites, which react with hemoglobin, displacing oxygen and resulting in a bluish appearance of the skin. If medical treatment isn't provided, the infant can die of asphyxiation.

Is Your Tap Water Safe?
Here's How to Find Out

"Drink plenty of water" is the advice often given by many health experts. But what do you do if you question the quality of your drinking water?

You can have your water tested by a professional or with one of the many do-it-yourself kits, or you can send samples away to a testing company. (See Additional Resources at end of this chapter.) But the results you get *today* may be different from the results you get *tomorrow,* because most municipal water treatment plants use chlorine to disinfect bacteria in water and the amount of chlorine remaining in the water changes from day-to-day or even from hour-to-hour depending on the original condition of the water. Also, since many systems get their water from more than one source, the results of tests taken on one particular day could be startlingly different the next.

What you *can* do is get some specific information about the types of water pollution that usually occur in your area. Look on your water bill to obtain the name and phone number of your water supplier. Whether it is a government body or a private company, it will have "customer relations" or "public information" employees. Call them.

Under the Safe Drinking Water Act (amended in 1986), all citizens have the right to obtain the following information about the drinking water from their local water supplier:

- What is its source?
- How is it treated to remove bacteria and other contaminants?
- What contaminants has the drinking water been tested for?
- Have contamination levels been found that violate current federal or state drinking water standards?
- What contamination problems have existed in the past and what exist currently?
- How has the public been notified about the violations?

Furthermore, the Safe Drinking Water Act of 1974 gives you the following protections:

- You have the right to bring civil suits against your local water system, or your state or federal officials if they fail to do their job. Civil penalties of up to $25,000 per day can be assessed by the courts depending on the seriousness of the violation and the danger to public health.
- The public water system is required to chemically treat contaminated water or install clean-up equipment to remove the contaminant(s) to below certain standards when a violation occurs.
- Major contaminant violations (those above certain concentration levels) must be publicly stated within 14 days of their detection and these notifications must occur at least once every three months if the contamination continues. These public notices should include a clear explanation of the violation, notice of potential adverse health effects, and explanation of the steps being taken to correct the problem.

Serious Health Threat to Your Family: Lead-Contaminated Water

Scientists estimate that lead in drinking water affects 4 million children yearly, contributing up to 20 percent of the total lead that young children are exposed to. The federal government confirms that figure and says the risk of lead poisoning is greater than previously believed. We will discuss other sources of exposure to lead in the next chapter, but we focus on the health dangers of lead-contaminated water here.

"The main and profound effect of lead is on the children. It causes impairments in reading, writing, mathematics, abstract thinking, and concentration span—all the skills necessary for academic success."

Dr. John Rosen, chairman of a committee advising the Centers for Disease Control.

Because they absorb more of any lead that they ingest and because of their small body size, children are more sensitive to the effects of lead; thus they are more likely to be harmed by lead in drinking water than are adults. Long-term exposure to low levels of lead may cause a buildup in the brain and other tissues resulting in slower growth, behavioral disorders, and decreased intelligence. An 11-year study by Dr. Herbert L. Needleman, M.D., a professor of psychiatry and pediatrics at the University of Pittsburgh, found that children who had moderate lead exposure when young had greater absenteeism from school, impaired reading skills, and were seven times less likely to graduate from high school than classmates who had little or no exposure.

"Young adults have a seven times higher rate of not graduating from high school and a six times higher rate of reading disability after early childhood lead exposure."

Herbert Needleman, M.D. in New England Journal of Medicine.

Epidemiological and experimental evidence indicates that children's risk of developmental problems is increased when their blood levels of lead are as low as 10 to 15 micrograms per deciliter or more. At least four million preschool children in the United States had blood levels exceeding 15 micrograms per deciliter in 1991, according to the Centers for Disease Control and the Agency for Toxic Substances and Disease Registry.

EFFORTS TO REMOVE LEAD FROM WATER   In 1986, Congress passed a set of amendments to the Safe Drinking Water Act of 1974; these amendments banned the new use of lead pipe and lead solder in public drinking water systems. Yet, in 1991 the EPA reported that half of all the public utilities in the United States still deliver water to homes through lead pipes installed in previous years.

Many historians believe that the Roman Empire fell because too many of its citizens became sick from lead exposure. One source was their water supply. (Another was contamination of their wine from lead-lined utensils.) In response to this same type of threat, in 1991 the EPA set what it calls the world's strictest rules for lead in drinking water—but it gave cities up to 21 years to correct their lead problems!

The EPA will soon mandate that public water systems monitor lead levels at high-risk homes. The new monitoring program is to begin in 1992 for municipal systems serving more than 3,300 people. The EPA set "action levels" for lead content in municipal water at 15 parts per billion (ppb). Under these new rules, at least 90 percent of monitored household drinking water cannot have lead levels exceeding 15 ppb.

PROTECT YOUR FAMILY FROM LEAD CONTAMINATION IN WATER
Experts agree that you should have your children and your water tested for lead. Samples of tap water taken by the EPA in 580 cities in 47 states indicate that 16 percent of the water from U.S. kitchens contains 20 micrograms or more of lead per deciliter of water. That's 25 percent higher than the new maximums allowed by law.

In 1991, the federal government finally decided that all young children should have their blood tested for levels of lead. The testing should be available, at a minimal cost to parents, through your county health department.

How to Interpret the Results of These Tests. In October of 1991, the federal government issued the following guidelines:

- If, after testing, a child is found to have 20 micrograms or more of lead, the child should immediately be seen by a physician. The physician may prescribe nutritional and/or medical treatments to reduce the lead burden carried by your child. (Household water also should be tested for the presence of lead, and parents should consider lead eradication measures explained in the next chapter. Also consider lead eradication measures if your child is in one of the following categories.)

- Children with levels of 15–19 micrograms should be screened frequently to ensure that levels do not increase. Parents should receive nutritional and educational counseling to learn how the right diet might help prevent damage from lead to their children's health.

- Children with levels between 10–14 micrograms should also be frequently screened for lead levels in their blood. Below this range, the guidelines make no recommendations for intervention, partly because laboratory tests are imprecise in being able to measure lower levels of lead in blood. However, the CDC does recommend community-wide prevention activities in areas where many children have levels of 10 micrograms or more.

Before October 1991, the Centers for Disease Control had set 25 micrograms of lead per deciliter of blood as the threshold at which a child would be considered lead-poisoned. But then new scientific studies revealed that levels as low as 10 micrograms can be harmful.

How much is 10 micrograms? It's such a tiny amount that it is difficult to make comparisons to any unit of measurement that average people use. For example, a gram is about $\frac{1}{28}$ of an ounce; a microgram is one-millionth of a gram, so it takes 28 *million* micrograms to equal an ounce.

To guard against lead-contaminated water, take advantage of the federally mandated tap water monitoring program. If you suspect a problem with lead in your home, contact your municipal water supplier and ask to be a part of the program. If at least 10 percent of the monitored homes exceed the goal of 15 ppb, the public water system is required to adopt corrosion control measures to reduce lead. The corrosion control measures include ultimately replacing water service pipes made of lead that connect water mains and individual homes. However, as stated before, the municipalities have up to 21 years to implement the most stringent of these measures. And, if less than 10 percent of the monitored homes exceed the 15 ppb goal, then your public water supplier need do nothing.

Even if your public water system delivers lead-free water to your home, what actually comes out of your tap may not be lead-free. Since it was legal to use lead pipe, solder, and fixtures in the construction of private homes until 1986, your most likely source of water-borne lead exposure is your own home's plumbing.

According to the EPA, older homes almost certainly contain lead-pipe plumbing. Newer homes with copper pipes aren't necessarily safe, especially in homes that use water softeners. The reason is that the otherwise safe copper plumbing was installed using lead solder. The water softener can make the water more corrosive, slowly eating away at metal pipes. This loosens the lead solder in the joints causing it to leach into the water. A water softener installed at the point of use prevents this problem.

And don't forget water at your child's school. Tests done in one county in Florida on 71 drinking fountains in 36 schools found lead levels above 20 parts per billion, and kitchen sinks in 28 schools had high lead levels in water from their faucets.

SPECIAL PROBLEMS FOR RURAL HOME DWELLERS If you live in a rural area, you'll probably have to bear the cost of testing for lead-contaminated water yourself. It's best to use a state laboratory or a private lab certified by the state. Contact the government water pollution expert in your state (see Directory A) for a list of state-certified laboratories, or contact the EPA's Safe Drinking Water Hotline for a list of state-certified testing laboratories. Costs range from $20 to $75 each to test water samples.

Safe Drinking Water Hotline:
800-426-4791

Check your water pipes to see if they are made of lead, especially if you own an older home. Lead plumbing is dull gray, unlike copper or galvanized pipe. When a lead pipe is hit with a metal object, the resulting sound is a dull thud; hitting pipe made of copper, brass, bronze, or galvanized steel gives a ringing sound. If you have lead pipes, it's probably best to replace them. Of course this can be expensive. Your decision will probably hinge on the lead levels in your water and whether you have children in the home. If you do replace lead pipes, have your water tested for lead *again*. If lead is still found in your water, ask your water supplier to adopt corrosion control measures to prevent the lead from reaching your home. Your water supplier can add calcium, phosphate, or silica-based corrosion inhibitors at the water treatment facility to promote the formation of protective coatings inside pipes and plumbing throughout the entire water supply system until the problem is solved.

Legally, public water suppliers have up to two years to install initial lead-prevention water-treatment measures and another 12 months to do follow-up tests. Then they have to take further action within the 21 years. Thus it's likely to take some time to remove all lead from your water supply. In the meantime, if any lead at all is found in your tap water, take the following steps:

- Have all family members take tests to reveal levels of lead in their bloodstreams. If high levels are found (above 10 micrograms per deciliter), consult with your doctor about medical measures to reduce the contamination.

- Avoid drinking hot water from your taps since heat makes lead more soluble in water.

- Use cold water for all cooking for the same reason.

- Especially in the morning, run tap water a couple minutes before drinking it (running the tap pushes out water that had been sitting in the pipes for hours).

- If babies are in the home, flush the pipes using the above procedure before preparing infant formula or other feeding preparations.

- Use bottled water for drinking and cooking, and use tap water for everything else.

WARNING ON SCHOOL WATER

The on-again, off-again use of water in schools can cause lead levels to climb. "Water that remains stagnant in interior plumbing during weekends and vacations, or even from the close of one day to the beginning of the next, is in longer contact with lead solder or pipes, and thus may contain higher levels of lead."

Environmental Protection Agency (from St. Petersburg Times*).*

Protect against Chloroform

Chloroform, one of the cancer-causing organic compounds, is part of a chemical family known as the trihalomethanes. These substances are found in minute amounts in most chlorinated tap water. Chlorine is used widely by municipal water systems as a disinfectant. As such, it is a beneficial additive. The problem occurs when hot, chlorinated water, such as for hot showers, hits the air and chloroform is released. "Half the chloroform is released before the water hits the tub," says Lance A. Wallace, Ph.D., of the EPA's Office of Research and Development. He is the EPA environmental scientist who conceived and designed pioneering studies called the Total Team Assessment Methodology (TEAM). According to the TEAM studies, chloroform is also released from hot water used to wash clothes and dishes. The concern is that years of such exposure to chloroform increases a person's susceptibility to lung cancer and respiratory diseases.

The solution to the chloroform problem in bathrooms and kitchens is to increase ventilation by using vented exhaust fans or opening windows. Unvented, filter-type fans would just spread the chloroform around in the air.

Well Water Pollution

The EPA estimates that 10 percent of the nation's community drinking-water wells and four percent of rural domestic drinking-water wells have detectable residues of at least one pesticide. Also, more than half of the nation's wells contain nitrates, with about 1.2 percent of the community wells and 2.4 percent of the rural wells showing levels above 10 ppm, the maximum contaminant level established to protect human health.

Nitrates are formed in nature as part of the *nitrogen cycle,* the circulation of nitrogen and its compounds: Nitrogen in the air passes into the soil, where it is changed to nitrates by soil bacteria. Some nitrates are absorbed by plants, which are eaten by animals. Decaying plants and animals, and animal waste products, are in turn acted on by bacteria, and the nitrogen (gas) is freed for recirculation. However, not all the nitrates are absorbed by plants. Some seep deeper into the soil, finally coming to rest in groundwater aquifers that supply drinking-water wells. Also, nitrates from decomposing manure at dairy farms and feedlots and from septic tank seepage get into the soil and cause nitrate contamination of well water. Another source of contamination is from nitrates used in agricultural and lawn fertilizers. What isn't used by plants, seeps down into the water table.

PROTECT AGAINST CONTAMINATED WELL WATER   First, find out where your water comes from. Be particularly suspicious if it's drawn from a private well, that is, a well that you own or one owned by an individual or company that sells water. Private wells tend to be shallow and thus vulnerable to whatever has been dumped on the ground in the past. Many small communities pump water from wells that have been contaminated by pesticides or by nitrates.

A strong chemical taste or smell is a reliable indicator of severe contamination, but water can taste and smell good and still be contaminated. Most chemical pollutants don't smell or taste bad when diluted to a few hundred millionths or billionths of their full strength. The only way to be assured of safe water is to have it tested.

Some states have programs to analyze individual household water supplies at no cost or at a modest cost to the homeowner. States that do not have such programs often have a designated agency to refer you to a commercial lab that will test for a wide variety of contaminants. Such tests can be costly; a scan for two or three dozen of the most commonly found industrial chemicals can run approximately $150 or more. Most local health departments will at least test for bacterial contamination.

Also check for too high concentrations of minerals such as fluoride, zinc, and copper. Too much copper and zinc can give water an off-taste. Too much iron and manganese also produce an unpleasant taste, discolor plumbing fixtures, and stain laundry. Fluoride protects teeth against decay, but ultrahigh levels of fluoride in well water can contribute to osteosclerosis (hardening of the bones). The *Journal of the American Medical Association* reports a case of an Oklahoma woman whose osteosclerosis was traced to the high fluoride concentrations in her well—concentrations that were more than seven times the recommended intake level.

RADON IN WELL WATER   If you get your water from a well or a small community water system linked to wells, the water that is piped into your house may carry another deadly invader—radon.

"In some parts of the country, radon in well water can be a significant contributor to elevated levels of indoor radon," states the EPA.

The radon becomes airborne when the water is drawn up
through pipes and is agitated as it pours into sinks, tubs, and appliances. Thus simple household activities that use water, such as showering and washing dishes or clothes, can cause significant releases of
waterborne radon into indoor air. You're protected, however, if you
get your water from a large municipal system since radon is released
while the water is being treated in the system.

Protect your family from radon in well water. First, test your air for
radon levels (see Chapter 2). If the test canisters reveal radon levels
higher than you care to expose your family to, then consider testing
your water.

The experience of the EPA is that "as a rule of thumb" there
will be about one picocurie per liter (pCi/L) of radon in the home
for every 10,000 pCi/L of radon in the water. "Consequently, a
waterborne radon level of 40,000 pCi/L can result—by itself—in
an indoor air level of about 4 pCi/L," the level at which the EPA
recommends that radon remedies be considered.

Some states have programs to analyze radon in household water
and others don't. See Directory A to locate a government contact
in your own state. In states that do not have such programs, the
designated agency will probably be able to refer you to a commercial
lab that will analyze the results of a water sample from your home
for approximately $20 to $35. Often these firms will supply test
kits. Because the way in which a water sample is collected is very
important in obtaining a true radon measurement, follow directions
on the test kit carefully. If the initial water test indicates that you
may have a radon problem, do a follow-up test to verify the results.

If these tests show a significant amount of the radon coming
from your household water supply, you have two choices: remove
the radon from the air after it has left the water, or remove the radon
from the water before it gets into your indoor air.

To remove radon from the air, make sure the house is well ventilated near the points of water usage: the kitchen, laundry room, and
bathrooms. Where radon levels are low, good ventilation of bathrooms, laundry, and kitchen may be adequate to prevent the buildup
of radon in your home.

The second solution is to remove the radon from the well water prior to use. The simplest way is to store the water until most of the radon has gone through its natural radiation decay process. However, as the decay process takes several days this calls for a very large storage tank.

Other removal methods are based on the natural tendency for radon to be released when water is exposed to the air. Home aeration systems have been developed that spray the water through an air-filled chamber. A fan then moves the radon-contaminated air from the chamber to the outside. Such systems can be expensive, however, costing up to $2,500.

Radon levels in water can also be reduced by granular activated carbon (GAC). Typical GAC systems cost about $1,000 to $2,000. The system works because radon tends to become attached to activated carbon particles. If enough granular activated carbon is contained in a tank through which the household water flows, up to 99 percent of the waterborne radon can be captured. However, as the radon and other radioactive elements such as uranium are collected and build up, the GAC can produce exposure and disposal problems.

The ability of GAC to remove radon will be affected by the level of radon in the well water, the amount of water used per day, and the type and amount of other contaminants in the system. The EPA says that a typical GAC tank that holds $1\frac{1}{2}$ to 2 cubic feet of carbon can serve a family of four and reduce a waterborne radon level of 100,000 pCi/L down to only 10,000 pCi/L.

GAC devices are simple to operate and maintain and should last for years. The only routine maintenance required is replacement of a prefilter cartridge or rinsing out a permanent prefilter. (Because granulated carbon is a very fine material, it will filter out many small particles such as iron and other sediments in the water. Thus, if the GAC bed is not protected with a prefilter installed between the well and the GAC unit, the GAC bed would eventually clog.) See the drawing *Typical GAC installation.*

The placement of the GAC unit is very important since it can cause direct radiation exposure to you and your family. It should be placed far away from living areas. Outside the home is best, but locate it in an area where children won't be tempted to play. Shielding the tank with concrete or other radiation absorbent materials can reduce radiation levels, but add to total costs of the system. A

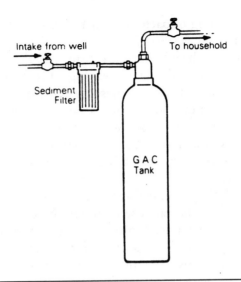

Typical GAC installation. (*Source:* EPA.)

knowledgeable dealer and your state or local radiation health office (see Directory A) can give you advice about using shielding.

Eventually the granular activated carbon bed will need to be replaced and the old carbon will need to be disposed of safely. Check with your state radiation control officer for advice on the proper way to dispose of it. If you can't find a listing in Directory A under your state, call the EPA regional office closest to you (see Directory B).

Devices to Clean Your Water

If you find your water contaminated by a specific pollutant and if the problem cannot be handled promptly by government sources, you may decide to install some sort of water purification device in your home. There are over 500 manufacturers of devices that purport to clean water. Most of these devices fall into three categories:

Activated Carbon Treatment Systems trap certain contaminants in charcoal filters. Like the radon-trapping carbon beds just mentioned, they are effective in trapping many volatile organic chemicals and industrial solvents as well as lead and certain pesticides. There are many types of carbon filters ranging from small (practically useless) units that screw on the end of a faucet to whole-house systems that attach to the water main. The latter systems require periodic maintenance to prevent the breeding of bacteria in dirty filters. Whole house units cost approximately $1,500 to $2,500.

Distillation systems heat water into steam and then cool the steam until it condenses back to water—leaving volatile and nonvolatile chemical contaminants behind. These systems also remove heavy metals such as cadmium, chromium, iron, and lead in addition to arsenic, nitrate, and sulfate. Used with a carbon filter, these systems produce the purest water possible. Distillation systems range from $225 to $1,500, and some are small enough to fit on a countertop or under the sink.

Reverse-osmosis (R-O) units force water through a membrane that filters out impurities. They are useful in removing arsenic, cadmium, chlorine, chromium, iron, lead, nitrate, radium, and sulfate and parasites such as *Giardia lamblia,* a protozoan that inhabits the intestines of various animals. However, most reverse-osmosis units use two to three gallons of water for every good gallon produced. The rest goes down the drain. The units are installed under the sink; costs range from $250 to $1,000.

Is Bottled Water Better?

Sales of bottled water are increasing faster than sales of any other beverage in the United States. One out of every 15 households now use it as the primary source of drinking water. Although many consumers buy bottled water because they like the taste, many others use it because of concern about the safety of their tap water.

Before spending a good deal of money on bottled water, make sure you know what you are buying. When buying bottled water, you may not necessarily have any more assurance of its safety than you do of the safety of water that flows from your own tap. Even though it's true that standards of quality for bottled water are at least as stringent as those for tap water, it's also true that 25 percent or more of bottled waters are little more than packaged tap water. There's nothing illegal about a company selling water it has gotten from a public supply. However, if you are paying a premium for what you think is "natural" or "spring" water, you may be disappointed. Read labels on the water bottles to determine the source of the water you are purchasing. If the label notes that the water is from a natural source or spring source, you can generally rely on that being true. If, however, it says "drinking water" or "bottled drinking water," then the water source is most likely a municipal water supply. Of course, if you believe the company's water supply source is safer than your own, it's perhaps worthwhile to buy such water. Water bottled from a public water source is generally less expensive than water labeled "natural," "spring water," or "purified." (See box for explanation of these terms.) You can also buy distilled water or water that has been processed by reverse osmosis.

If you do choose to purchase bottled water, check to see that the company that is packaging the water is a member of a trade group known as the International Bottled Water Association (IBWA). Also look for the term "NSF-certified" on bottle labels. Most IBWA members undergo a yearly unannounced plant inspection by the National Sanitation Foundation to make sure that standards at least as stringent as those for tap water are being met. Not all IBWA members are NSF-certified.

Defining Bottled Water Labels

- *Distilled water* is water that has been vaporized and recondensed. In the process, it is completely demineralized.

- *Purified water* is water that has been either distilled or processed by reverse osmosis.

- *Mineral water* is any undistilled water. All natural water has some minerals in it. However, the International Bottled Water Association defines its mineral waters as water that "contains not less than 500 parts per million total dissolved solids."

- *Natural water* is water that does *not* come from a public supply such as a municipal water system and has not been modified by the addition or deletion of any minerals. It can come from wells or springs.

- *Spring water* flows out of the earth on its own, unlike well water, which has to be pumped. It usually is unmodified by the addition or deletion of minerals and thus is often labeled "natural spring water."

- *Sparkling waters* (sometimes called seltzers) are waters that are either naturally carbonated or to which carbon dioxide has been added.

- *Club soda* is water that has been injected with carbon dioxide and to which salts and minerals have been added.

Just as municipal water providers can make mistakes, so can these commercial suppliers. *Consumer Reports* magazine in a recent investigation found that some bottled waters contain up to three times as much arsenic as is allowed by law. Even Perrier®, the so-called king of bottled waters, can produce contaminated water: Approximately 160 million bottles of Perrier were recalled during the summer of 1990 after traces of benzene were found in Perrier. Such a large-scale recall does, however, indicate a reassuring concern for providing a quality product. In the final analysis, only you can make the decision whether purchasing bottled water is best for your family.

The Safe Drinking Water Act's Failed Promise

In spite of all the concern about the safety of the public water supply, the EPA maintains that Americans enjoy one of the safest water supplies in the world. Undoubtedly this is true. Whether it's safe *enough* is still the subject of heated controversy.

When the Safe Drinking Water Act became law in 1974, Congress envisioned a major overhaul of the nation's drinking-water system. The legislation called on the EPA to determine what substances were contaminating our water, assess the potential health effects, establish legal health limits, and intervene where the states failed to enforce them.

Obviously the EPA has failed to live up to its mandate. For years the EPA had guarded our water against only the known threats—some 30 contaminants including microorganisms, nitrates, lead, and some organic chemicals. Finally, in response to the new knowledge and concern about water contamination, the EPA has set stricter drinking water standards for some substances and regulated other substances for the first time. The EPA now has established standards for 83 contaminants including such varied pollutants as dry-cleaning compounds, gasoline, fuel oil, solvents, degreasers, benzene, vinyl chloride, and carbon tetrachloride. It also has set stricter rules on the amount of lead that can remain in our drinking water.

Whether the new rules will do any good is also a subject of debate. The General Accounting Office (GAO), an investigative arm of Congress, says that there is massive noncompliance with the Safe Drinking Water Act (SDWA) and that the nation's more than 34,000 public water systems tally an average of about 97,000 violations per year. For the new rules to have the bottom-line result of keeping our water clean, they must be enforced. Yet enforcement breaks down at every level—local, state, and federal. In 1990, for instance, one in five water suppliers violated a health standard or didn't adequately test water. James Elder, the EPA's relatively new drinking water chief, admits that "48 to 49 states" are failing to adequately enforce existing regulations. Unfortunately, the EPA rarely intervenes, taking enforcement steps against only a small percentage of the most chronic offenders. As a result, the EPA has been actively criticized by Congress, the GAO, and environmentalists for failing to enforce drinking water regulations.

Quick Summary

Water is essential to life, yet most of us take safe drinking water for granted. However, nationwide water supplies are being polluted by chemicals and microbiological contaminants. You have to take the responsibility to ensure clean water in your home.

Flulike symptoms such as gastrointestinal upset and diarrhea may be caused by a variety of factors, but if many family members and neighbors have the same symptoms, it's a good idea to have your water tested.

It's also a good idea to have your water tested for radon and lead. If your water is contaminated, there are many steps, depending on the contaminant, that your water supplier should take, and many actions you can take to ensure the safety of your water. For example, you may want to install your own water-cleaning system or purchase bottled water until your water supplier "cleans up its act."

ADDITIONAL RESOURCES For information about pesticides and other contaminants that might be polluting the water in your locality call The National Pesticide Telecommunications Network (800-858-7378) and the Citizens Clearing House for Hazardous Waste (703-237-2249).

If you have only a rough idea of what you need to test for, you may want to test for an assortment of contaminants. Tests for numerous contaminants usually cost about $200. Three national laboratories with efficient delivery systems for picking up water samples anywhere in the country are WaterTest (800-426-8378), Suburban Water Testing (800-433-6595), and National Testing (800-458-3330). For further information on testing laboratories, write: American Association for Laboratory Accreditation, 656 Quince Orchard

Rd, Gaithersburg MD 20878; or call 301-670-1377; or the American Council of Independent Laboratories, 1629 K Street NW, Washington DC 20006; or call 202-887-5872.

If you decide to purchase a water purification system, be aware that dealers who are certified by the Water Quality Association (WQA) may be more reliable than uncertified dealers. For a list of WQA-certified dealers, write WQA, 4151 Naperville Road, Lisle IL 60532; or call 708-505-0160.

For more information on bottled water write: International Bottled Water Association, 113 N Henry St, Alexandria VA 22314.

For other information on water call the EPA's Safe Drinking Water Hotline at 800-426-4791 or write: Clean Water Action, 1320 18th Street NW, Third Floor, Washington DC 20036.

For information on well water write: American Groundwater Trust, National Well Water Association, 6375 Riverside Dr, Dublin OH 43017 or call 800-423-7748.

CHAPTER **9**

PERILOUS PAINT

The Hidden Hazard Posed by Paint

In August of 1989 a previously healthy four-year-old Michigan boy was diagnosed with acrodynia, a painful, rare manifestation of mercury poisoning. He suffered excruciating leg cramps, rash, itching, swelling, excessive perspiration, rapid heartbeat, weakness in his lower legs, intermittent low-grade fevers, headaches, hypertension, and redness and peeling of his hands, feet, and nose. Doctors discovered high levels of mercury in his urine. Following four months of hospitalizations and intensive rehabilitation, most of the young boy's symptoms faded, but he still has weakness in his legs.

He was lucky. In 1991 a 28-month-old boy in Wiaukesha, Wisconsin, died after eating chips of lead-based paint. According to Wisconsin epidemiologist Joe Shirmer, who investigated the case, the boy's death "was a dramatic example of the worst-case scenario of what happens if paint is ignored as a source of lead exposure."

In this chapter we will examine the dangers posed by paint additives, especially those posed by mercury and lead.

Mercury Pollution

No less a historic personality than Isaac Newton is said to have been affected by mercury poisoning. Historians note that Newton's personality changed dramatically when he was 35—he became irritable, paranoid, and withdrawn—and again when he was 51, after experiments involving heated mercury. It is thought that he inhaled the dangerous fumes. Indeed, in modern times English scientists who

141

analyzed a lock of Newton's hair found unusually high levels of mercury.

Both mercury and lead come from numerous sources. A ubiquitous source of both substances is paint. Until 1990, many latex paint manufacturers added mercury as a fungicide to their paints.

HEALTH DANGERS OF MERCURY Mercury poses many dangers to health. According to Barbara Scott Murdock, editor of *Health & Environment Digest,* some of the severe effects of mercury vapor poisoning in adults include: "personality disturbances, trembling hands and eyelids. Other symptoms include gingivitis, loose teeth, blindness, deafness, and damage to the cerebellum [leading to loss of equilibrium]." Whereas such effects often stem from chronic, relatively high exposure, even low-level exposures are of concern.

Low-Level Exposure to Mercury is a Concern to Scientists

"Our present concern about mercury vapor stems from effects of low-level exposures. These include subtle effects on the nervous system such as short-term memory loss, slight tremor, and effects on kidney function."

Thomas Clarkson, Ph.D., University of Rochester Environmental Health Sciences Center.

Mercury vapor poses a special hazard to children because it is heavier than air and tends to accumulate on the wall close to baseboards where crawling infants can inhale it. Thus small children are more at risk than adults.

However, researchers investigating the Michigan case mentioned earlier found that the boy's only exposure to mercury was from paint applied to the interior of his home ten days earlier. This prompted an epidemiologic survey by the Centers for Disease Control (CDC), which compared 19 Michigan homes that had been recently painted with a brand of paint containing mercury with ten homes that had *not* recently been painted with a mercury-containing paint. Residents of the 19 exposed homes had higher amounts of mercury in the air of their homes than residents of the ten comparison homes. Eighty-eight percent of the residents allowed their urine to be tested. Those living in homes painted with mercury-containing paint had higher levels of mercury in their urine than the comparison group.

"Mercury compounds in paint are volatile enough to raise the total indoor air mercury concentration by 1,000 times the level present before the paint is applied," said Dr. Mary M. Agocs, who headed the team of epidemiological researchers. Her team of researchers speculated that after the paint was applied and as it dried, the mercury vaporized and was released into the home environment, where it was inhaled by residents.

There was enough evidence from the CDC study for paint and mercury manufacturers to agree to voluntarily stop adding mercury to interior latex paint after August 20, 1990. Although paint companies voluntarily agreed to cease the use of mercury in the paints they manufactured after that date, the problem has not been completely solved because there has been no federal recall of mercury-contaminated latex paint. Because of this irresponsible shirking of federal responsibility, stocks of paint that were produced prior to August 20, 1990 are still on many store shelves and, depending on the turnover in any particular store, could remain on the shelves for years to come. Since there are 1,600 different brands of latex paint that might contain mercury, there are too many to list in this book. However, if you have purchased a paint that might have been manufactured before August 20 of 1990, you can call the National Pesticide Telecommunication Network at 800-858-7378. That number is a toll-free line jointly maintained by the EPA and the Agency for Toxic Substances and Disease Registry (ATSDR). The latter agency is the federal public health agency charged with "preventing or mitigating adverse human effects and diminished quality of life resulting from exposure to hazardous substances in the environment." When you call the hotline, a consultant will check the name and lot number of the paint you have purchased on their computer data base and tell you whether the latex paint you have is likely to contain mercury.

IF YOU HAVE ALREADY USED A MERCURY-CONTAINING LATEX PAINT
Experts aren't sure how long homeowners should be concerned about mercury emissions from painted walls. We talked to one such concerned expert, Dr. Barry L. Johnson, an assistant Surgeon General and assistant ATSDR administrator, who told us: "It appears that mercury outgasing occurs for at least seven or eight months. Some researchers tell me it could take as long as five to seven years for the mercury in some latex paints to outgas, but there is

adequate information to state that conclusively." (Outgasing is the process by which a solid substance emits into the air gaseous molecules of its chemical substance.)

"We're not sure what the lowest safe level for mercury exposure is," warns Dr. Thomas Clarkson of the University of Rochester Environmental Health Sciences Center. "Mercury may be like lead— in that for prenatal exposures even very, very low levels may cause delayed development in young children."

> "Chronic low-level mercury vapor exposure may affect concentration and short-term memory. Long-term health effects may include low I.Q., nervousness, and allergy."
>
> *Minnesota Department of Health.*

HOW TO GUARD AGAINST THE DANGERS OF MERCURY IN PAINT

- Check the manufacturing date of any latex paint and, if in doubt, call the National Pesticide Telecommunication Network.

- Whenever you paint, open windows and provide as much ventilation as possible. Proper ventilation of affected areas both during and after painting will do much to alleviate the problem.

Lead Pollution

The problem of mercury-based paints pales in comparison to that of lead-based paints. Before 1950, lead was routinely added to paint. Even though concerns were raised in the 1950s and 1960s, the addition of lead to paint wasn't banned until the 1970s. Paint high in lead content had the advantage of continuous chalking, thereby providing renewed surfaces and a long-lasting, fresh look. However, the sloughing off of paint particles created a serious public health danger.

"The greatest source for childhood lead poisoning is not old pipes, but old paint," stated the CDC. One of nine children under age six has enough lead in the blood to be placed at risk, says the Department of Housing and Urban Development (HUD). The housing agency also says that 57 million homes in America built before 1980 contain 3 million tons of lead-containing paint.

> "The fact is that lead poisoning is now being called the nation's no. 1 environmental threat to children—not by Greenpeace or Ralph Nader, but by top officials of the Bush administration."
>
> Newsweek, July 15, 1991.

HEALTH DANGERS AND SYMPTOMS OF LEAD POISONING   In children, exposure to lead-based paint can retard mental and physical development and reduce attention span. In adults, high doses of lead can cause fatigue, irritability, poor muscle coordination, and nerve damage in both sensory organs and motor nerves. Lower-level lead exposure may also cause problems with reproduction and may increase blood pressure. Often symptoms don't appear until the lead poisoning reaches dangerous levels, and if there are early symptoms, they are easy to confuse with other illnesses. Early symptoms may include persistent tiredness, irritability, loss of appetite, stomach discomfort, reduced attention span, insomnia, and constipation. The problem is even worse if the person also has a deficiency of calcium, zinc, or especially iron since such deficiencies result in increased gastrointestinal absorption of lead.

> "Lead exposure has already cut in half the number of U.S. children who might have had superior I.Q.'s (125 or higher)—some two million kids."
>
> Herbert Needleman, M.D., Professor of Psychiatry and Pediatrics, University of Pittsburgh.

IS YOUR HOME SAFE?   Most homes built before 1980 should be tested. Seventy-four percent of all private housing built before 1980 contains *some* lead paint. About two-thirds of the homes built before 1940 and one-half of the homes built from 1940 to 1960 contain *heavily* leaded paint. Leaded paint may have been applied on any interior or exterior surfaces. It often is found on woodwork, doors, and windows. To be safe, consider having the paint in your home tested for lead if it was built before the 1980s, especially if the paint or underlying surface is deteriorating or if you plan renovations. Don't wait for symptoms to occur. If you have children who live in a house that has been painted with lead-based paint, it is vital that you have them tested for lead levels in their blood. Most local health departments maintain free or nominal-cost screening programs. In children, the current blood lead level that defines lead poisoning is 10 micrograms of lead per deciliter of blood. However, extremely susceptible individuals can be affected at even lower levels. Adults usually don't need to have their blood levels tested for lead unless they have experienced exposure to lead through renovation of the home or unless they exhibit lead exposure symptoms.

CHILDREN ARE ESPECIALLY AT RISK Although the ban on lead paint has been in existence since the 1970s, the presence of lead in older housing poses a serious hazard, especially to small children. The CDC and the U.S. Public Health Service in a joint statement say: "Lead poisoning remains the most common and societally devastating environmental disease of young children. . . . We now know that large numbers of children may suffer adverse health effects at blood lead levels that were once considered safe."

Particularly worrisome are the latest scientific findings that relatively low-level lead exposure in children can result in delayed learning, impaired hearing, growth deficits, and adverse behavioral effects.

"One of the most sensitive targets of lead and other toxic metals in our environment is the developing brain."

Bernard Weiss Ph.D., Environmental Health Services Center, University of Rochester School of Medicine, Rochester NY.

Once thought to be a medical problem mainly for low-income families living in run-down, older homes, lead poisoning is now known to be a widespread problem for all economic groups. Consumers at all income levels can be exposed to lead-based chalks, chips, or peels from deteriorated surfaces.

So don't take it for granted that your home is safe because your income allowed you to purchase an average or better-than-average house; "1.8 million homes [contaminated by lead] are occupied by children whose families have incomes above $30,000, which is approximately the median income for all households," says HUD in a 1990 report to Congress. Furthermore, the CDC and the U.S.

Public Health Service warn: "We have made little progress in eliminating lead-based paint in older homes as a cause of childhood lead poisoning."

> "Lead-based paint is the source of greatest public health concern. Most children with lead poisoning are never identified."
>
> *Strategic Plan for the Elimination of Childhood Lead Poisoning, developed for the U.S. Department of Health and Human Services.*

A Victim of Lead Poisoning Speaks

Monica Santiago, 15, was diagnosed as having lead paint poisoning in 1979. She has been in special education programs throughout her school years. As a plaintiff in a legal action filed in federal District Court in Boston against producers of lead pigment that had been added to the paint, she was quoted by the *New York Times* as saying: "I want to be a lawyer, but I don't think I can do the studying. In school they teach me, but I forget. The kids call me dumb. Sometimes I get mad or sad and don't know why. My tears fall fast."

Monica's lawsuit was one of the first filed against the producers of lead pigment added to paint. Hers is one of many filed in state and federal courts against not only manufacturers of lead-based paint but also the producers of lead pigment.

[handwritten annotation: Different common places where you find hazard]

HOW LEAD GETS INTO THE BODY One way young children are exposed to lead is by eating paint chips. It doesn't matter that you may have taught your children not to eat paint chips. Children are attracted to lead-based paint chips because they taste sweet.

Adults too are at risk. For instance, opening or closing a painted frame window can create lead dust that can be inhaled. Removing old, lead-based paint or knocking down walls or home renovations that generate lead dust can cause lead poisoning in adults.

If your home was painted with lead paint, the soil around it may be contaminated, and lead-contaminated dust and soil can be tracked into the home. Residents can be poisoned by inhaling this dust. Infants and crawling children often put their hands to their mouth and thus eat paint chips.

Middle and upper-income families are as likely to have lead paint in their homes as the poor. Children of lower, middle, and upper-income families can be exposed to the dangers of lead poisoning during the renovation or restoration of older houses. You, and the workers you hire, can generate lead dust by sanding, scraping, or heating lead-based paint. The lead can enter the lungs and get on the skin. Lead dust settles on floors, walls, and furniture, making it easy for children to ingest by hand-to-mouth contact. Vacuuming or sweeping may raise the lead dust into the air again, where it can be inhaled.

One such case was reported in the prestigious *American Journal of Public Health*. Mr. and Mrs. A and their children, a five-year-old daughter and a 20-month-old son, moved into a Victorian farmhouse in rural upstate New York in late June of 1987. They hired workmen to renovate the old house. By mid–October they noticed their ten-year-old dog "shaking and twisting." She was taken to the family veterinarian, who found her to be dehydrated and weak. It turned out that the dog "had developed a fondness for one of the workmen and sat by his feet while he sanded old paint. She was often seen licking her dusty coat." The dog soon died of kidney failure brought on by lead poisoning.

The dog may have saved its owners' lives. They too were experiencing symptoms. Mrs. A reported she had been feeling tired and weak. Her daughter had complained of stomachaches. Mr. A had had an episode of severe nausea after spending a weekend at home while renovation work was proceeding. All three were found to have high blood levels of lead. All underwent a treatment known as chelation therapy to remove lead from their systems. Chelation is the use of certain chemicals to remove an excess of heavy metals such as lead from the bloodstream. Sometimes chelating formulas are given orally and sometimes intravenously. Although improved, Mrs. A still felt weak and tired. A pregnancy test was performed and she was found to be eight weeks pregnant. She decided on a therapeutic abortion because of the high chance that the fetus would have mental or other congenital defects from the lead. The authors of the *American Journal of Public Health* article wrote:

> Many old homes are undergoing restoration today by new owners. Sanding, torching, and the use of heat guns to remove the old layers of paint are common. These methods produce chips, fine dusts, and fumes that can be ingested or inhaled. Lead fumes, which are

generated by heat removal, using either torches or blowers, are especially dangerous because they produce small, easily respirable particles less than one micron in diameter.

Exposure to such particles or lead fumes can produce acute lead poisoning within days or even hours.

LEAD IN DINNERWARE   According to the American Academy of Pediatrics, lead-glazed pottery is another potential source of lead in food and drink. If not fired at high temperatures, lead may be released from the glaze in large amounts when such pottery is used for cooking or for storage of acidic foodstuffs. Also, if pottery vessels are washed frequently, even a properly fired glaze can deteriorate, releasing unsafe levels of previously adherent lead.

Among the oldest sources of lead in America is antique pewter. Food should not be cooked or stored in antique pewter vessels or dishes. Although uncommon, many of these sources have been associated with severe symptoms and even fatal lead poisoning.

There may also be lead in the foil caps on your wine bottles, put there to keep rodents in wine cellars from chewing on the corks. Advice: Use a damp cloth to wipe the rim and neck of the bottle before serving.

WAS MY HOME PAINTED WITH LEAD-BASED PAINT?   Although there are do-it-yourself lead testing kits available, none have been evaluated by the U.S. Consumer Product Safety Commission. Many of these tests give false-positive results; however, they can still serve as a screening mechanism to indicate whether you have lead-based paint in your home. Don't panic if you get a high reading. It just means you need to do more sophisticated testing.

Cure

Here are two do-it-yourself lead testing kits that can be used to do initial lead paint tests, according to the consumer health magazine *In Health*. The kits have passed the muster of the Consumers Union, and cost close to $30.

The Frandon Lead Alert Kit   Leadcheck Swabs
Frandon Enterprises   HybriVet Systems, Inc.
511 N 48th St.   P.O. Box 1210
Seattle WA 98103   Framingham MA 01701
800-359-9000   800-262-LEAD

The most reliable way to determine if you have a lead problem is to have a laboratory test paint samples from various areas of your home. Lab testing is more reliable and less expensive than another popular method, x-ray fluorescence, a method in which a technician comes to your home and uses an x-ray machine to scan your walls for lead paint. Lab tests of paint samples cost from $20 to $50 per sample. And you'll need to take multiple samples. A single sample from the living room might miss lead paint in the kitchen. Sample the paint of each suspect room. To get a sample for a lab test for lead paint, do the following:

- Use a sharp knife to cut off a paint chip at least two inches by two inches.

- Lift off the paint chip with a clean putty knife and put it into a resealable plastic bag. Make sure you get all layers of paint in your sample; however, don't include underlying wood, plaster, or brick.

- With a wet paper towel, wipe any paint dust off the surface where you took the sample, being careful not to get any into the air. Discard the paper towel.

- Repaint the scraped surface to seal off a potential source of lead paint dust.

SHOULD LEAD BE REMOVED FROM YOUR HOME? Should lead in the home be removed, thus risking the chance of increasing lead levels in the air, or should it be allowed to remain, perhaps covered up or sealed in some way? Each family's situation is unique. The problem of removing lead from homes is complex. If you try to remove it, you may increase your family's potential risk by causing lead particles to become airborne. Yet lead can be removed if proper safety controls are in place. We'll talk about these safety controls in a moment. The best advice we can give about removing lead is to consult with local experts (see Directory A for whom to contact in your own area) for advice as to whether it is necessary to get lead removed from your house. An important factor to consider is whether your family is being contaminated by lead. If you have high levels of lead in your home, family members should have yearly blood tests to monitor levels of lead.

ADVICE ON REMOVING LEAD PAINT The U.S. Department of Housing and Urban Development (HUD) recommends that action be taken to reduce exposure when the lead in paint is greater than 0.5 percent by lab tests. Remember, however, properly defusing a lead paint problem in a home is complex, dangerous, and likely to be expensive. The work done to remove lead-based paint can pose a danger in itself. Unless adequate cleanup is done, residents moving back into homes may be harmed by microscopic lead particles left behind. The best control methods are those that disturb the paint least. Sanding, dry scraping, and open-flame burning are not recommended because they create great amounts of hazardous dust and lead fumes.

Here are ATSDR's recommendations: _Cure_

- Often the best solution for lead-painted windows and doors is to replace them.

- On large surfaces such as interior walls or exterior boards, a process called encapsulation may work. This involves covering lead paint with a permanent sealing material, such as acrylic or epoxy coatings, that bonds to surfaces. Another method to make lead paint inaccessible is enclosure. For example, sheetrock can cover interior walls, and siding materials such as aluminum or vinyl can contain peeling or chalking exterior paint.

- To reduce lead dust exposure after the work has been finished and you have moved back in, use a high-efficiency particle accumulator (HEPA) vacuum cleaner, and periodically wet mop and wipe surfaces and floors with a high-phosphate (at least 5 percent) cleaning solution. Ask for trisodium phosphate (TSP) washes at paint or hardware stores. Wear waterproof gloves to prevent skin irritation.

- If you opt for having the lead-based paint removed, hire professionals trained in how to do this work safely. Be sure the professionals understand the importance of containing lead dust when they remove moldings, trim, window sills, and other painted surfaces. Have them wet clean the entire area before you move your family back in. It is extremely important to stay out of the house during both the days and the nights while the work is being done.

- A lead removal project on a standard three-bedroom home takes three to four weeks so prepare to spend time in temporary housing. The home should not be entered until samples of dust have been collected from walls and other surfaces and analyzed to

Turn

determine if the house is still contaminated. If lead dust remains, further cleaning is necessary.

LEAD PAINT TESTING AND ABATEMENT COSTS   Although each home is different, an ATSDR survey indicates that inspection firms charge owners of single-family homes anywhere from $300 to $1,500 for testing. Don't panic. HUD says the average cost is closer to $300 per home.

The cost of lead abatement depends on how much lead paint is in the house, the types of building components needing treatment, and the method of abatement used. If tests reveal high levels throughout the home, expect to spend anywhere from $5,500 to $12,000 for a contractor experienced in lead eradication. Actual costs will depend on what method of lead abatement is used and whether the home has an interior or exterior lead paint problem or both.

There are six different methods used to lessen lead hazards. Two methods (encapsulation and enclosure) work by isolating lead hazards and four other methods (chemical stripping, abrasive removal, hand scraping, and component replacement) permanently remove the lead from the dwelling.

The method that is often the least hazardous and least expensive, according to experts, is encapsulation—sealing off all sources of lead. By encapsulation we don't simply mean painting over lead-based paint with a nonlead paint. This isn't a solution because the lead-based paint will continue to loosen below the painted surface and will eventually escape to create lead dust. Even when lead-painted surfaces are properly encapsulated with an acrylic or epoxy coating, care must be taken to monitor these surfaces. At the first sign of wear, hazardous areas should be recoated.

It bears repeating: Before deciding on the best strategy for your home, consult with experts. To find a lead abatement specialist, contact your state or local health department's lead-poisoning prevention department or other helpful state governmental agencies such as housing authorities. This book's Directory A will be helpful in this regard. Be cautious, though. Remember that although specialists may be referred by a government body, they may not actually be credentialed by that body. Take the time to ask contractors about their qualifications and experience in removing or containing lead-based paint. *Money* magazine, in a July 1991 article, recommends that consumers hire a contractor who has had experience with at least a dozen separate lead eradication projects.

Lead Paint Removal Guidelines from the U.S. Department of Housing and Urban Development

- Keep children and others, especially infants, pregnant women, and adults with high blood pressure, out of the work area until the job is completed.
- Remove all food and eating utensils from the work area.
- Cover all cabinets and surfaces that come into contact with food and keep them sealed while the work is going on.
- Remove all furniture, carpets, and drapes, and seal the work area from the rest of the house. Have the contractor seal off the floor.
- Workers should not wear work clothing in other areas of the house.
- The use of heat guns to remove lead-based paint is *not* recommended. HUD says that the use of these tools puts high levels of lead dust into the air.
- Contractors should clean up debris using special high-efficiency particle accumulator (HEPA) cleaners, and wet mop after vacuuming.
- Contractors should dispose of lead-based paint waste and contaminated materials in accordance with state and local regulations.

What if you can't afford these measures and you think your old home might have lead-based paint? One expert said that, although inadequate, she would at least buy 5 percent trisodium phosphate and wipe down window casings and walls twice a year.

Another Danger from Indoor Exposure to Paint—Bis(Tributyltin) Oxide

The removal of mercury from paint has caused some owners to mix fungicide additives in paint to control the growth of fungi and mildew in the home. The problem is that some additives have been implicated in causing health difficulties. One such chemical is bis(tributyltin) oxide (TBTO), a tin extract that has been in use as a fungicide for many years. However, TBTO has been shown to cause weight loss, suppressed immune systems, and anemia in animal studies. In humans, skin exposure produces itching, redness of the skin, inflammation of hair follicles, eye and throat irritation, sore throat, and cough. These symptoms were dramatically illustrated in January 1991 when a pregnant Wisconsin woman contacted her local public health department to report that she and her two children had become seriously ill after her landlord painted the walls and ceilings of two rooms of her apartment with paint to which TBTO had been added.

Reported symptoms included a burning sensation in the nose and forehead, headache, nosebleed, cough, loss of appetite, nausea, and vomiting. The woman, who was in the third trimester of her pregnancy, and her two children were removed from the apartment. One day after moving out, one of her children was treated in a hospital emergency room for persistent vomiting. The other child developed a persistent cough, but did not require medical attention. Eight days after moving out of the apartment the woman gave birth to a healthy infant. However, over the next 12 weeks she had to take the child to a pediatrician several times for evaluation of persistent vomiting, rashes, and respiratory difficulties. The woman had recurrent burning pain in her nose and forehead for at least three months after exposure. Both of her older children reportedly recovered without persistent symptoms. Two days after the family moved out of their apartment (nine days after the painting) the Wisconsin State Health Department measured an air sample from one of her bedrooms and found there was still a significant amount of TBTO in the air.

Wisconsin health officials could have benefited from similar earlier experiences in the state of Washington. In 1988 Washington's Department of Health issued a health advisory warning against using TBTO in interior paint. The warning was based on the state's investigation of six incidents of illness among persons who painted one or more walls or ceilings with interior paint to which this fungicide had been added. Yet most states, including Wisconsin, had still not issued such advisories even as this book went to press. Most states don't have mechanisms set up to receive reports of paint or paint additive-related illnesses.

Because such illness-reporting mechanisms don't exist in most states, Lynden Baum, the public health specialist who co-wrote the Washington State health advisory, believes the reported cases may be harbingers of larger numbers of adverse reactions to come.

"There's considerable potential for harm because TBTO additives are sold nationwide. Some states require such products to be labeled 'for exterior use only' but many don't even require that warning. This is unfortunate because most homeowners don't understand the potential hazards."

Added Dr. Mark McClanahan: "What they do understand is that they have fungus or mildew growing on an interior wall and when they repaint they want to add something to retard its growth." Mc-Clanahan is a health scientist at the National Center for Environmental Health and Injury Control. He too believes that reported cases are just "the tip of the iceberg. Considering the widespread availability of these products, the potential for harm is great."

TBTO additives are sold in paint stores under many brand names including ADD-X®, Biomet®, and Super Di-All Mildewcide®. The EPA has no policy mandating a warning against adding TBTO to interior paint, but the agency is now advising homeowners not to add TBTO to interior paint, according to Dr. Carl Grable, an EPA plant pathologist and spokesperson for the EPA on that issue. TBTO is added to exterior paint by paint manufacturers, but such paints carry warnings that the product should only be used on the exterior of homes.

Quick Summary

Paint may hold many hidden health hazards including mercury, lead, and TBTO poisoning. The health effects of poisoning from these sources can be temporary or permanent and can range from eye, nose, and throat irritation to death. Children are especially at risk.

ADDITIONAL RESOURCES *Comprehensive and Workable Plan for the Abatement of Lead-Based Paint in Privately Owned Housing: A Report to Congress,* by the U.S. Department of Housing and Urban Development (HUD), December 7, 1990. Send $3.00 to HUD User, P.O. 6091, Rockville MD 20980. For detailed guidelines on lead removal that your contractor should follow, write Alliance to End Childhood Lead Poisoning, 600 Pennsylvania Ave SE, Suite 100, Washington DC 20003.

The following articles provide excellent background. They are available in libraries:

- "Mercury: An Indoor Air Pollutant," an article by Ruth A. Etzel, M.D., and Mary M. Agocs, M.D., in *Health & Environment Digest,* May 1990, vol. 4, no. 4.

- "Mercury Exposure from Interior Latex Paint," an article by Mary M. Agocs, M.D., Ruth A. Etzel, M.D., et al., *The New England Journal of Medicine,* October 18 1990, pp. 1096–1101.
- *The Nature and Extent of Lead Poisoning in Children in the United States: A Report to Congress,* by the Agency for Toxic Substances and Disease Registry, U.S. Department of Health and Human Services, Public Health Service, July 1988.
- *Strategic Plan for the Elimination of Childhood Lead Poisoning,* published February 1991 by the U.S. Public Health Service and the Centers for Disease Control.
- "A Case Report of Lead Paint Poisoning during Renovation of a Victorian Farmhouse," by Phyllis E. Marino, M.D., Philip J. Landrigan, M.D., M.S., et al. in the *American Journal of Public Health,* October 1990, vol. 80, no. 10.
- "Acute Effect of Indoor Exposure to Paint Containing Bis(tributyltin) Oxide—Wisconsin, 1991," in *MMWR—Morbidity and Mortality Weekly Report,* May 3 1991.

CHAPTER 10

TOXIC THREATS

Potentially Dangerous Products and
Hazardous Wastes in the Home

In 1991, nine-year-old David H of Denver developed a set of bewildering, life-threatening symptoms: stomach pain, vomiting, diarrhea, and a high, unexplained fever that lasted for days.

Doctors suspected strep throat, scarlet fever, hepatitis, or an
unidentified virus. They were wrong. David had developed symptoms of a rare affliction known as Kawasaki syndrome probably as
a result of being exposed to freshly shampooed carpeting. Scientists speculate that some chemical in the shampoo produced David's
life-threatening symptoms. In fact, fifty percent of all Kawasaki syndrome victims come down with the affliction after being exposed
to freshly shampooed carpets, but the brands of shampoo vary and
scientists haven't yet identified the chemical or combination of chemicals at fault.

David, however, was lucky. Doctors finally made the right diagnosis and his life was saved. But many others are at risk—about
1,000 North American children under the age of five are stricken by
the disease each year. About one in 50 of these children die.

David's case is an extreme example of what can happen when
we are exposed to chemicals used routinely in the home. Americans
and citizens of other industrialized societies use and store in their
homes a bewildering array of chemical substances. The EPA lists
more than 50,000 different chemicals in general use, although fewer
than 2,100 have been tested for immediate or long-term side effects.
Add the potential plethora of chemicals used by people for cleaning, deodorizing, disinfecting, exterminating, painting, polishing,
and personal grooming to the 4,500 possible constituents of tobacco

smoke and it's no wonder that the air quality of our homes is often an unhealthy "witch's brew."

Exposure to indoor air pollutants translates into lost productivity, ill health, and major annoyance to 75 percent of the population, according to many experts. That's three out of four of us! The odds are, you are affected.

. In response to this indoor air quality problem, one state has appeared as a leader. In 1991, California adopted the nation's toughest air-quality standards for household products. The standards, which are being phased in from 1993 to 1998, will cut smog-forming pollutants by 45 percent from such products as aerosol hairspray, window cleaner, and floor wax. Other products covered by the tough new regulations include engine degreaser, windshield washer fluid, furniture polish, room air freshener, laundry prewash, nail polish remover, insect repellent, oven cleaner, hair-styling gel and mousse, tile cleaner, and shaving cream.

Organic (carbon-based) chemicals are widely used as ingredients in products such as those listed above. Many cleaning, disinfecting, cosmetic, degreasing, and hobby products contain organic solvents, as do paints, varnishes, and wax. When you use these products, they release possibly harmful chemicals and organic compounds into the air you breathe.

In 1990 more than 30,000 children under 6 years of age drank hydrocarbons in the form of kerosene, lighter fluid, turpentine, gasoline, furniture polish, paint thinner, naphtha, or typewriter correction fluids.

From Contemporary Pediatrics, *December 1991.*

Defining *Poisonous,* *Toxic,* and *Hazardous*

Chemicals play a vital part in our lives and most of them are not dangerous to our health or the environment, if used and disposed of properly. Too often people think of chemicals as "poisons." *Poisons* are chemicals that produce illness or death even when taken in very small amounts. Whereas not every chemical is a poison, every chemical is inherently toxic at some level. However, that doesn't mean that every chemical, at any concentration, is hazardous.

Toxicologists, those scientists who study the effects of chemicals, have found it useful to give special meanings to the terms *toxicity* and *hazardous*. In a nutshell, *toxicity is the inherent property of a chemical to produce a damaging effect when the chemical has reached a sufficient concentration at a certain site in the body.* The concept of *hazard* is more complex, writes Dr. M. Alice Ottoboni, a California toxicologist and author of the book, *The Dose Makes the Poison: A Plain-Language Guide to Toxicology.*

> The hazard presented by a chemical has two components: one, the inherent ability of a chemical to do harm by virtue of its explosiveness, flammability, corrosiveness, toxicity, etc., and two, the ease with which contact can be established between the chemical and the object of concern.

Thus an extremely toxic chemical such as the poison strychnine, when sealed in an unopenable container, can be handled freely by people with little or no hazard. It is still *toxic,* yet presents no *hazard* because no contact can be established between the poison and people.

There are two types of toxicity: *acute* toxicity and *chronic* toxicity. The acute toxicity of a chemical refers to its ability to do damage to the body or its functioning as a result of a *one-time exposure* to a relatively large amount of the chemical. For example, acute toxicity is of concern when children are exposed to certain household products left carelessly within their reach. Acute effects are of overriding concern when considering indoor air pollution issues. Chronic toxicity, on the other hand, refers to the ability of a chemical to cause health effects as a result of *many repeated exposures* over a prolonged period of time to relatively low levels of the chemical.

Chronic toxicity is the major reason why the plethora of chemical products mentioned earlier is of concern. We are all subject to repeated exposures to low levels of many chemicals, often for prolonged periods of time. Individual exposures may not cause adverse health effects, but *cumulative exposure* may result in a *threshold* effect at which we become sick. Different people have different thresholds to individual chemicals.

Besides the threshold effect, there's the question of the adverse health effects a person might experience when exposed to more than one chemical contaminant at a time. The EPA warns that when several chemical contaminants are mixed together the combination could potentially cause adverse health effects "at levels below thresholds presently known to cause adverse health effects." That means that shorter exposures to small amounts of several chemicals may cause adverse health effects quicker than might be expected if we are exposed to just one chemical at a time. That's what may have happened to David. His exposure to several chemicals in the rug shampoo may have triggered his life-threatening symptoms. Why David and the other 999 children who react with Kawasaki syndrome each year were more sensitive to these chemicals than youngsters who didn't become sick is not known.

The Air You Breathe May Be Hazardous to Your Health

Lance A. Wallace, Ph.D., is the EPA environmental scientist who in 1980 conceived and designed a pioneering, ongoing study that measured personal exposure to a wide range of environmental pollutants in more than 2,000 people who lived in or around 12 U.S. cities. The results were eye-opening: For most pollutants in the study, *the air outside may be safer to breathe than air inside the home!*

Whether they live in a rural area or in a city, many homeowners are exposed to an amazing amount of chemical pollutants, says Wallace, explaining that most people's exposure to known or suspected cancer-causing chemical pollutants appears to come primarily from personal activities in the home. His study identified polluting activities such as smoking, showering, storing and wearing dry-cleaned clothing, and using cleaning and deodorizing products. Quoting the comic strip *Pogo,* Wallace says, "We have met the enemy and he is us."

His quote refers to the fact that our choice of lifestyle condemns many of us to living with high levels of indoor air pollution. It's a matter of choice. Your neighbor may have dramatically lower indoor air pollution levels than you do—especially if the neighboring family has broken its chemical habit while your family remains hooked on aerosol spray products such as room deodorizers, furniture polish, and hair-styling preparations.

Desserend common places

DANGER OF ROOM AIR FRESHENERS AND MOTH REPELLENTS   Room air fresheners and moth repellents are prime examples of modern-day products that are indoor air-polluting villains. Many air fresheners and moth repellents (whether they are mothballs or moth-repelling cakes) contain a chemical named para-dichlorobenzene (P-DCB) as a main ingredient. It is one of the most potent cancer-causing agents in the home. When inhaled in high concentrations by humans, it can cause headaches, nausea, and mental confusion. Dr. Wallace says that P-DCB is "almost exclusively an indoor air pollutant. According to some estimates it poses the highest cancer risk of all indoor chemicals studied in the last decade. Well over 90 percent of personal exposure to this chemical comes from deodorizer and mothproofing preparations."

Incredibly, manufacturers of room air fresheners and mothproofing preparations aren't required to list their ingredients. One product, Enoz Moth-Ice® crystals by Willert Home Products says the following on its label: "Warning: California has determined that a chemical contained in this product causes cancer based on tests performed on laboratory animals." The product also carries this statement: "Precaution. Hazard to humans and domestic animals. Harmful if swallowed. Avoid contact with skin, eyes, or clothing." The precaution says nothing about possible dangers from inhalation.

DRY CLEANING CHEMICAL DANGERS   Another source of indoor air pollution are the clothes we bring home from the dry cleaners. Tetrachloroethylene, the solvent usually used for dry cleaning, has been proven to cause cancer in animals. EPA studies have shown that "garments recently dry-cleaned are the major source of personal exposure to tetrachloroethylene." In fact, dry cleaning accounts for 90 percent of all the tetrachloroethylene we are exposed to; whereas other household sources, such as paints, solvents, and cleansers such as spot removers and carburetor cleaners account for the remaining 10 percent of total exposure.

THE VOLATILE ORGANIC COMPOUNDS   The chemicals just discussed belong to a large class of chemicals known as volatile organic compounds (VOCs). They are organic (carbon-based) chemicals that evaporate readily at room temperature. The EPA studies found that the average levels of VOCs were at least two to five times higher inside homes than outside regardless of whether the homes were located in rural or highly industrial areas. (Individual homes can have levels 100 to 1,000 times higher than outdoor levels for an individual VOC.) Those VOCs that are typically found in high indoor concentrations include:

- Tetrachloroethylene from dry-cleaned clothes and degreasers.
- Chloroform from chlorinated water.

- Benzene from tobacco smoke, gasoline fumes, and power mower or automobile gasoline evaporations in attached garages.
- Formaldehyde from fabrics, pressed wood products, insulation, and cosmetics.
- Styrene found in adhesives, foam, lubricants, plastics, carpets, and insulation.
- Methylene chloride from paint strippers.
- Para-dichlorobenzene (P-DCB) from deodorizers and moth repellents. Although these products don't list specific ingredients, many aerosol air fresheners do note what percentages of their contents are made up of VOCs. For instance, the label on Airwick® states that it contains 23% VOC, Renuzit® states 38% VOC and Wizard® states 46% VOC. Air deodorizer "sticks" or solid "cakes" and most moth repellents don't usually even give that much information.
- Carbon tetrachloride from paint removers and dry-cleaning preparations. Once commonly found in cleaners, spot removers, and paint removers, carbon tetrachloride is considered pound for pound more destructive of the ozone layer of our atmosphere than even the well-published chlorofluorocarbons (CRCs). Because of its cancer-causing potential, it has been removed from household products yet still can be found in stocks of old products.
- Trichloroethane from pesticides, spray can propellants, insulation, photographic equipment, and spot removers. A recent store shelf survey found it in a Dow product called K2R Spotlifter®, labeled with the following warning:

  Caution: contains perchloroethylene and trichloroethane. Do not treat garment while wearing. Do not spray in eyes or on skin. If contact occurs, flush thoroughly with water. Avoid prolonged breathing of vapor. Do not puncture. Do not throw in fire as container will burst. Exposure to temperatures above 120°F may cause bursting. Do not use near fire or flame. Intentional misuse by deliberately concentrating and inhaling contents can be harmful or fatal. Keep away from children.

Health Dangers of Volatile Organic Chemicals

The health effects of VOCs vary widely. Some are highly toxic in relatively small concentrations, whereas others have few health effects even at high concentrations. Acute health effects from low-level exposures include eye, nose, and throat irritation, fatigue, visual disorders, headache, nausea, dizziness, and even impaired memory and depression. Some people experience problems with their vision and suffer memory impairment almost immediately after being exposed to some of these organic chemicals. More frightening are the potential long-term effects. Many organic compounds—such as formaldehyde, chloroform, trichloroethylene, and tetrachloroethylene—are known to cause cancer in animals and are suspected to cause cancer in humans. Some, such as benzene and methylene chloride, *are known to cause cancer in humans.* Let's take a closer look at the sources and dangers of three of these chemicals.

TETRACHLOROETHYLENE   Also known as perchloroethylene, this is the chemical most widely used in dry cleaning. It has been shown that this chemical causes cancer in animals and that people breathe low levels of this chemical when dry-cleaned clothes are stored in the home. To minimize exposure, when you bring dry-cleaned clothes home, hang them outside to air out. Don't be fooled if you can't smell a chemical odor. You are still being exposed. Hang them on a porch or at least by an open window away from the living areas of your home for at least 12 hours.

BENZENE SOURCES AND HEALTH DANGERS   Among the most prevalent VOCs found in homes is the chemical benzene. It is found in tobacco smoke, in stored fuel and paint, and in automobile emissions that enter the home from attached garages. Benzene is a known cause of leukemia. It also causes eye and respiratory tract irritation, headaches, dizziness, and visual disorders.

You can reduce benzene exposure by eliminating smoking within the home, providing maximum ventilation during painting, and by discarding (or moving them away from the house) leftover paint supplies and special fuels (such as charcoal lighter) that will not be used immediately. If possible, do not park your car in an attached garage. If you have to park in a garage attached to your home, do *not* idle the car's engine in the garage because exhaust can thus enter the home.

Several years ago when the EPA's Dr. William McClenny was testing the accuracy of new air-monitoring equipment in dozens of homes, he discovered that his own Raleigh, North Carolina home had the highest chemical levels of all. All it took to fix his problem was a little effort. Dr. McClenny moved his lawnmower and his gas, oil, and paint cans from his basement and garage to an outside storage shed. When he again tested his home's air a few months later, most of the chemicals from the first reading were significantly reduced.

METHYLENE CHLORIDE SOURCES AND HEALTH DANGERS A "Consumer Product Safety Alert" has been issued by the U.S. Consumer Product Safety Commission (CPSC), on the organic compound methylene chloride. (See the illustration titled *Methylene chloride health hazards.*) Methylene chloride is a colorless, volatile, nonflammable liquid with a penetrating, ether-like odor that has been found to cause brain and nervous system damage as well as cancer in rats. This chemical causes cancer in some laboratory animals and may pose a cancer hazard to humans. Methylene chloride is converted to carbon monoxide in the body and can cause impaired vision and coordination, headaches, dizziness, confusion, and nausea as well as fatigue and flulike symptoms and chest pain in people with heart conditions.

The CPSC warned people to not use the following products indoors and not to breathe the vapors. At least some (but not all) products in the following categories contain methylene chloride:

- Spray primers and aerosol spray paints for autos
- Adhesives and glues and their removers
- Cleaning fluids and degreasers
- Glass frosting and artificial snow
- Spray paints, paint thinners, and paint strippers
- Spray shoe polish
- Water repellents
- Wood stains and varnishes

In a recent survey of store shelves in several U.S. cities conducted by University of Alabama journalism students, the following brand names were found to contain methylene chloride: Dad's™ Easy Spray, Formby's Paint Remover®, Gillespie Old Furniture Refinisher®, Glidden's Revised Goof Off Blend®, Klean Strip Paint Remover®, and Klean Strip X Creamy Paint Stripper® as well as Klean Kutter Remover®; Kwikeeze Water Rinsing Brush Cleaner®, Nasco

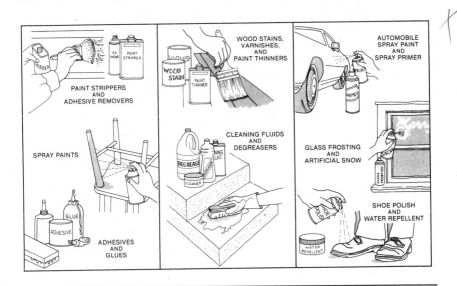

Methylene chloride health hazards. (*Source:* CPSC, September 1987.)

Sandpaper in a Can®, Permatex Disk Brake Quiet™ and Permatex Gasket Remover®; Savogran® Kutzit Paint and Varnish Remover, Silicone Tire Shine®, Strypeeze® Paint Remover, and Strip X™ Paint Remover.

Warning labels vary, but a typical variation was: "Health hazard information: Contains methylene chloride, which has been shown to cause cancer in certain laboratory animals; risk to your health depends on level and duration of exposure." Another warning read: "Danger Poison, extremely flammable. May be fatal or cause blindness if swallowed. Vapor harmful, skin and eye irritant." In smaller print, below the warning label was the following: "Read other cautions and health hazard information on back panel." On the back label, it stated that reports on methylene chloride have shown that "associated repeated or prolonged occupational overexposure to solvents may cause permanent brain damage and nervous system damage."

Many products, such as Formby's, include a toll free number (800–FOR-MBYS), which customers can use to ask questions about the product. The customer representative who forthrightly answered our call acknowledged the cancer risk and encourages callers to provide adequate ventilation when using the product and, if doing a large amount of paint stripping, to break the job up into intervals so as not to be exposed to dangerous vapors continuously for hours.

One's risk depends on both the level and duration of exposure. To reduce exposure, use products that contain methylene chloride outdoors. If a product containing methylene chloride must be used indoors, open all windows and doors, and use a fan to expel the air outside during application and drying. The CPSC warns that harmful exposure can occur even without immediate or observable symptoms such as headaches, dizziness, and watery eyes.

A CPSC warning in 1987 (shown in the illustration) caused many companies to reformulate their products. For instance, Scotchgard® for Cars; Derusto®, a rust-preventive enamel; and Elmer's® Slide All adhesive remover have notices on their labels proudly boasting that they contain *NO* methylene chloride.

Even though products containing methylene chloride are now supposed to be labeled with warnings, many manufacturers may be using substitute substances in the same chemical family—halogenated hydrocarbons. These substitute chemicals may be used as ingredients in everything from shoe polish to tire cleaners, but there may or may not be warnings to consumers. The most commonly used of these halogenated hydrocarbons is a substance known as 1,1,1-trichloroethane. This VOC with a strange-looking name is often found in household cleaners, spray can propellants, pesticides, and in dry-cleaned clothes. It's in hundreds, possibly thousands of products. A recent survey of store shelves found it in several products including CRC Brakleen®, Elmer's® Contact Cement, Gila® Spray Film, Snap® Silicone Tire Shine, Super-X® Brake Cleaner, and DURO® Contact Cement. The DURO product listed this warning: "Caution: Vapor and liquid are harmful. Contains 1,1,1-trichloroethane. Avoid prolonged or repeated breathing of vapor or contact with eyes. In case of eye contact, flush thoroughly with water and get medical attention. Use only in well ventilated area. If swallowed, do not induce vomiting. Call physician immediately. Keep out of the reach of children."

The reason for the warning is that 1,1,1-trichloroethane is recognized as a "toxic" substance. Although not considered a possible cancer causer, acute (one-time) exposure can cause people to become sick. Some authorities also worry that cumulative exposure to this chemical can cause a threshold effect resulting in damage to the central nervous system or other organs.

THE FEDERAL GOVERNMENT IS LAX ABOUT POSSIBLE DANGERS
There are many other chemicals in household products that medical authorities worry about, but about which not enough is known,

especially regarding their cumulative or combined effects. Federal government agencies seem to be lax in financing and releasing the proper studies and then following up with regulative actions. For instance, in 1991 the EPA finally released results of a study entitled "Indoor Air Pollutants from Household Product Sources." The study was actually a reanalysis of information on the chemical contents of 1,159 household products done originally in 1987. The original research had identified the six common chlorocarbons in household products including methylene chloride and substitute solvents such as 1,1,1-trichloroethane. Four years later the EPA finally reexamined the data on 25 additional chemicals found in those products. Those chemicals "found most frequently in household products," according to the 1991 reexamination included acetone, which was in 315 products; 2-butanone, 200 products; toluene, 488 products; methylcyclohexane, 150 products; m-xylene, 101 products; and o,p-xylene, 93 products. In high-concentrated doses, toluene and the xylene chemicals have been found to cause liver and kidney problems and adverse central nervous system effects. The other chemicals also have been shown to cause assorted adverse health effects in test animals and sometimes in humans. 2-butanone, for instance, in high concentrations has been implicated in causing incapacitating fatigue of workers in an office building.

Are these chemicals being used in commercial products? And if so, what is being done? The answer to the first question is: almost certainly. Yet neither the EPA nor the CPSC really knows, since it was four-year-old data that was being reanalyzed. Since the manufacturers have been under no pressure to reformulate, it's likely that the chemicals remain.

What is the CPSC doing about the situation? Apparently nothing. When asked about the potential problem of halogenated hydrocarbons, a top CPSC source expressed concern only about the adverse health effects of the xylenes.

How to Protect Your Family from Household Chemicals

Obviously, concerned home-dwellers can limit their exposure to potentially toxic substances by not purchasing the products containing suspect chemicals. However, not all products are well labeled or give a complete listing of ingredients. Some products, for instance, just list ingredients as "halogenated hydrocarbons." (For example,

Helmsman® Spar Urethane by Minwax says it contains "halogenated hydrocarbon 30.")

If you must use such products, the following steps will help you reduce exposure to potential harmful household chemicals.

HOW TO HANDLE TOXIC HOME PRODUCTS

- Carefully follow label instructions. For example, if a label says to use the product in a "well-ventilated" area, go outdoors or to areas equipped with an exhaust fan to use the product. Or open windows.

- Do not store unneeded chemicals. Later in this chapter we explain how to rid your home of partially full containers of old or unneeded chemicals. Because gases can leak even from closed containers, this one step can do much to lower concentrations of organic chemicals in your home.

- If you must store chemical products, make sure that they not only are stored in a well-ventilated area but also are kept safely out of the reach of children.

- Buy limited quantities of toxic products. Buy only as much as you will use right away of products such as paint strippers, kerosene for space heaters, or gasoline for lawnmowers.

**Two Common Toxic Product
Mistakes in Homes with Children**

- Are cleaning products stored on countertops and window ledges or on the floor or bottom shelves of low cabinets without safety latches? Move them out of reach of a curious child. Install safety latches.

- Check the bathroom. Is the toilet bowl cleanser kept on the floor behind the toilet and the tub cleanser kept on the bathtub ledge? Move them onto a high place out of reach of a small child.

How to Choose Nontoxic, Environmentally Safe Home Products

You can replace hazardous household products by making or buying safe "green" or "nontoxic" ones. *Green* is a term that originated in

Europe, where it initially described policies and actions that were environmentally friendly. Today it is being used by advertisers to proclaim that products are environmentally sound both in packaging and contents. Be warned though: The terms, *green, nontoxic, natural,* and *environmentally safe* have no universally accepted or legal definitions. Most over-the-counter detergents, bleaches, and polishes sold in supermarkets are manufactured from toxic chemicals such as hydrochloric acid, sulfuric acid, and benzene. Be skeptical if you see those ingredients in products that are supposedly "environmentally safe" or "nontoxic."

Here are basic guidelines of what to look for both in terms of packaging and in terms of what's inside.

- Whenever possible, choose items packaged in paper, cardboard, glass, or aluminum rather than plastic.

- Buy larger sizes of products to cut down on packaging.

- Try to purchase products in refillable containers.

- Buy unbleached, recycled, or chlorine-free products. (Traces of dioxin, a chemical that may cause cancer, have been found in a variety of paper products at potentially harmful levels. Dioxins are created in the paper-making process when pulp is bleached to make paper whiter.)

- If you now use bleached paper coffee filters, switch to unbleached paper filters, washable cotton filters, or a reusable gold mesh filter to avoid possible contamination by dioxin.

- Instead of mothballs use cedar, an excellent nontoxic moth repellent. Cedar chips or blocks can be put in drawers and closets, trunks, or garment bags. Cedarwood boards are available from lumber supply companies. Cedar chips can be obtained at many garden and pet shops. Cedarwood oil and cedar blocks are available from catalog companies.

- Try to use household cleaning products that are biodegradable, or make them yourself. Avoid phosphate and petroleum products because they contribute to global pollution. Many companies now make biodegradable, petroleum-free soaps and cleansers, including Arm & Hammer®, All Free and Clear®, Bon Ami®, Ivory Snow®, and Fels Naphtha®. Baking soda, salt, and vinegar are also nontoxic, effective cleansers.

NONTOXIC CLEANING PRODUCTS

Disinfectants and drain cleaners. Disinfectants and drain cleaners are dangerous to both people and the environment, but you can make alternatives that are both nontoxic and nonpolluting. For instance, instead of commercial disinfectants, use one-half cup of borax in a gallon of hot water. To keep a drain from clogging, pour one-quarter cup of baking soda followed by one-half cup of vinegar. Close the drain until fizzing stops, then flush with a gallon of boiling water.

Bathroom. The best time to clean your shower is right after using it, when steam has loosened the dirt. Just wipe off damp surfaces with a sponge. You can remove mildew from a shower curtain by washing the shower curtain in a solution of bleach and water in your washing machine on its gentle cycle. You can use baking soda to clean sinks and basins.

Unpleasant odors. If there are unpleasant odors in your home, the first course of action is to open the windows and air out the house. If weather conditions don't permit this simple answer, use $\frac{1}{4}$ cup white vinegar and a drop or two of peppermint in a pump sprayer rather than a commercial air freshener that may contain formaldehyde. Or place containers of baking soda around the room to absorb unpleasant odors.

Window cleaners. To clean windows, use a solution of one cup of vinegar in a gallon of hot water. If you have streaking problems, add a small amount of rubbing alcohol into the vinegar and water solution.

Oven cleaners. To clean an oven, try this easy, two-step method that uses baking soda, salt, and hot water. First splash salt and hot water over greasy, grimy areas. Then sprinkle with baking soda and leave until morning. You'll be able to wipe off the grease and grime easily the next morning with a mildly abrasive pad. After all the grime is removed, use clean water to remove any baking soda residue.

Laundry stains. To remove wine stains, pour salt on them. To remove grass, tar, or oil stains, use eucalyptus oil. Fruit or tea-stained clothes can often be cleaned by boiling them in water. To get rid of perspiration stains on clothes, soak them in a mixture of water, baking soda and/or white vinegar. Lemon juice and salt are effective on rust stains. To bleach soiled white socks, soak in baking soda before washing or boil them in water containing a slice of lemon. Also white clothes can be hung out to dry, as sunshine bleaches whites.

Wood finishes. Instead of commercial furniture polish, use a mixture consisting of equal parts olive oil and white vinegar and a couple drops of lemon oil. Shake well. It will put a shiny protective gloss on cabinets and other wood surfaces.

Floor cleaners. For a superb floor cleaner, use one cup of white vinegar in a pail of water or one-half cup borax® to two gallons of hot water.

Disposal of Hazardous Wastes from the Home

One way to lower the amount of chemical indoor air pollution in your home is to get rid of old, potentially hazardous household chemicals. Thousands of household products contain ingredients that pose threats, not only to the air quality of your home but also to your children, because the products are caustic, corrosive, inflammable, chemically unstable, or perhaps even explosive. Even when properly stored and sealed, some of these chemicals can leach into the air. Any product that is several years old should be considered a candidate for removal.

But don't just throw these hazardous products into the trash. Experts estimate that one percent of America's household waste is potentially hazardous. If you throw toxic materials in with your regular trash, you add to the problem. Compacted in a garbage truck, most containers break, causing health danger to sanitation workers. When dumped in a landfill, the hazardous products will slowly leach into the ground and could ultimately contaminate drinking water.

Don't just pour hazardous products down the drain. Household drains flow to municipal sewers or septic tanks, which are not designed to handle hazardous wastes. Don't dump hazardous waste into storm drains; most storm drains dump their contents directly into streams, rivers, and oceans. You would just be polluting the earth.

Exactly how you should dispose of hazardous wastes depends on the individual substance and how your community treats trash. Some communities have drop-off sites for household hazardous wastes. Other communities set up special hazardous waste collection days. Check with your local government or private environmental organizations to see if your community sponsors special days for the collection of hazardous and toxic household wastes. If your

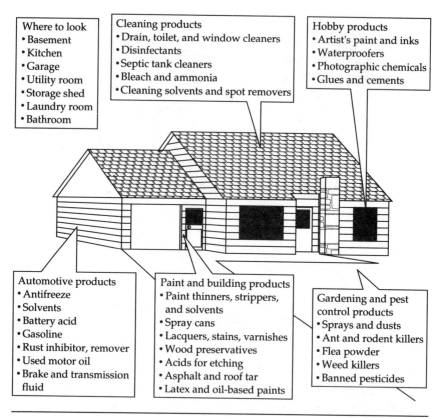

Where to look
• Basement
• Kitchen
• Garage
• Utility room
• Storage shed
• Laundry room
• Bathroom

Cleaning products
• Drain, toilet, and window cleaners
• Disinfectants
• Septic tank cleaners
• Bleach and ammonia
• Cleaning solvents and spot removers

Hobby products
• Artist's paint and inks
• Waterproofers
• Photographic chemicals
• Glues and cements

Automotive products
• Antifreeze
• Solvents
• Battery acid
• Gasoline
• Rust inhibitor, remover
• Used motor oil
• Brake and transmission fluid

Paint and building products
• Paint thinners, strippers, and solvents
• Spray cans
• Lacquers, stains, varnishes
• Wood preservatives
• Acids for etching
• Asphalt and roof tar
• Latex and oil-based paints

Gardening and pest control products
• Sprays and dusts
• Ant and rodent killers
• Flea powder
• Weed killers
• Banned pesticides

Hazardous wastes in the home.

community doesn't have such a program, consider organizing one. The League of Women Voters of Massachusetts makes available a video and a kit of materials on how to set up collection days for household hazardous waste products. For information, write to the League at: 8 Winter St., Boston MA 02108. Or call the EPA's RCRA/Superfund hotline at 800-424-9346 to order a free EPA publication entitled *Household Hazardous Waste: A Bibliography of Useful References and List of State Experts.* Also, experts in some states are listed in Directory A at the end of this book.

Some hazardous wastes can be made safe for collection. For instance, some aerosols, liquids, and paints can be safely disposed of by spraying them outside onto newspaper, cardboard, or into kitty litter. Allow the liquid contents to soak up and evaporate. The remaining newspaper, cardboard, or kitty litter can then be thrown away with regular garbage.

Here is a list of some potentially hazardous products in your home and how to dispose of them:

- *Pesticides in aerosol cans.* Whether empty or partially full, these should be put aside for collection and disposal in a hazardous waste facility.
- *Furniture polish.* If in an aerosol container, it can be emptied as described earlier by using the newspaper/kitty litter method.
- *Insect repellent.* If in an aerosol container, these can also be depressurized or sprayed out for evaporation.
- *Batteries.* Depleted household batteries should be dropped off at a hazardous waste facility.·
- *Nail polish remover.* These can be evaporated using the kitty litter/newspaper method.
- *Upholstery cleaners.* Check the label. If the contents are flammable or if it contains the cancer-causing solvent chloroethylene, the container should be taken to a hazardous waste facility. If it is water-based, it is safe to throw away.
- *Wood preservatives.* If you have old stocks of these chemicals, they may contain creosote or pentachlorophenol, hazardous ingredients banned for consumer use since 1985. Landscapers and plant nursery workers in most states have had training in how to use these products safely. They may be interested in taking them off your hands. If that is not possible, put them aside for a trip to the hazardous waste facility.
- *Household scouring powders.* They can be safely thrown into the trash.
- *Used automotive oil.* Many service stations will take used automotive oil for recycling.
- *Other automotive supplies (antifreeze, transmission fluids, hardened car wax).* Some automotive stores will accept labeled containers of old fluids for disposal. Your state highway department may be able to give you an address of an oil-recycling station that will take them. As a last resort, while outdoors, pour the fluids into a container of sawdust or cat litter, seal it and put it in the trash.
- *Partially used paints.* You might contact a charity or a local theater group to see if they need it for set decoration. You can dry out old latex or oil-based paint by leaving it outside in an open can and then discard in the trash.

- *Paint thinner or turpentine.* These should be sealed tightly in their original containers and taken to a hazardous waste disposal site.

Quick Summary

Many everyday household products contain toxins that endanger our health. Not all toxins are hazardous *if* they are handled properly. In fact, many toxins can be avoided entirely by buying environmentally safe ("green") products or by making your own cleansers and deodorants. Buying such products will reduce the total amount of toxic substances to which your family is exposed and has the added advantage of being less expensive. If you must purchase toxic products, be sure to buy only what you need, handle them properly, and keep them safely out of children's reach.

ADDITIONAL RESOURCES   The Consumer Product Safety Commission (CPSC) is investigating carpet-related health complaints. Their carpet study is part of the Commission's larger project on indoor air pollutants from products. Consumers who believe they may have suffered adverse health effects after the installation of new carpet or the use of other carpeting products should call the CPSC toll-free at 800-638-2772. For carpet complaints write: Carpet Complaints Room 529, U.S. Consumer Product Safety Commission, Washington DC 20207.

The American Lung Association of Delaware has free indoor air pollution brochures, including a fact sheet on household products. To receive information, write to them at: 1021 Gilpin Ave Suite 202, Wilmington DE 19806.

The Clean Air Council's Indoor Air Pollution Center has a complete library on causes of indoor air pollution. The Center can be reached by calling 215-545-1832 or writing them at: 311 S Juniper St Suite 603, Philadelphia PA 19107.

Other Resources (Publications and Articles)
- *Indoor Pollutants*, by the National Research Council, published in 1981 by the National Academy of Science Press.
- "Even Air in the Home Is Not Entirely Free of Potential Pollutants," *Journal of the American Medical Association*, December 8, 1989.
- *The Inside Story: A Guide to Indoor Air Quality*, by the EPA and the Consumer Product Safety Commission.

Sources of nontoxic household cleaning information

- For a list of natural cleaning alternatives, send $2 to the Clean Water Fund, 808 Belmar Plaza, Belmar NJ 07719. Also check the following books.

- *Cheaper and Better,* by Nancy Birnes, published in 1988 by Harper. Lists hundreds of homemade alternatives to commercial products.

- *Clean & Green: The Complete Guide to Nontoxic and Environmentally Safe Housekeeping,* by Anne Berthold-Bond, 1990, Ceres Press. Includes 485 ways to "clean, polish, disinfect, deodorize, launder, remove stains—even wax your car without harming yourself or the environment."

- *Favorite Helpful Household Hints—Clean, Fix, and Organize Your Home,* by the editors of *Consumer Guide.* Describes 4,000 tips.

- *Home Ecology: Simple and Practical Ways to Green Your Home,* by Karen Christensen, 1990, by Fulcrum Publishing, Golden CO.

- *The Nontoxic Home: Protecting Yourself and Your Family from Everyday Toxics and Health Hazards,* by Debra Lynn Dadd, published by Jeremy Tarcher, 1986.

- *Nontoxic, Natural, & Earthwise: How to Protect Yourself and Your Family from Harmful Products and Live in Harmony with the Earth,* by Debra Lynn Dadd, published by Jeremy Tarcher, 1990.

CHAPTER 11

ELECTROMAGNETISM

Should We Be Worried?

Can electromagnetic energy, generated by the transmission and use of electricity, cause cancer or other health problems? In a society that literally runs on electric power, the very idea that electromagnetic energy can be dangerous to health seemed preposterous at first. However, for more than a decade growing numbers of scientists have been doing studies that suggest a link between exposure to electromagnetic fields and increased risk of certain types of cancers. These researchers were originally ridiculed and charged with being alarmists, but recently their work has gathered new respect.

The issue was examined by the U.S. Environmental Protection Agency. In a draft report under review by an independent group of scientists and other experts as this book went to press, the EPA sounded its most serious warning to date on the subject. The report found that the "weight of evidence," including nine studies involving humans, "suggests a causal link" between extremely low-frequency electromagnetic (EM) fields and leukemia, lymphomas, and nervous system cancers.

What does a "causal link" mean? An EPA source told the authors: "With our current understanding we can identify 50–60 Hz electromagnetic fields from power lines and perhaps other sources in the home as a *possible, but not proven*, cause of cancer in people." The EPA position on EM fields, however, will not be formalized until scientific and public review of the draft report is completed.

The risk of leukemia among children with the highest exposure to magnetic fields is about two times greater than the risk of leukemia among children with the least exposure to EM fields, according to the most recent study on the subject. The five-year, $1.7 million investigation financed by the electric utility industry and conducted by the University of Southern California (USC) was published in the November 1, 1991 issue of the *Journal of Epidemiology*. The study was described by USC as being "the most comprehensive to date of childhood leukemia and exposure to electromagnetic fields." Researchers compared 232 Los Angeles County children who got leukemia by age 11 with 232 who did not. The researchers found that children with leukemia were more likely than healthy children to use 11 out of 15 electrical appliances. An elevated risk for leukemia was statistically significant for two appliances—electric hair dryers and black-and-white television sets.

Electromagnetic Fields Defined

What is electromagnetic (EM) radiation anyway? Visible light is an EM effect. You can read this book and otherwise enjoy the gift of vision because of EM radiation. Light is only one of many different forms of EM radiation. EM wave bands also include frequencies beyond those of human senses. Radio waves and x-rays are examples.

There are electric and magnetic fields wherever there is electric power. This means that electromagnetic fields are emitted by large and small power lines and by wiring in homes, workplaces, and all electrical appliances. Electric blankets, water bed heaters, and microwave ovens are particularly of concern, exposing you to relatively high EM field levels because they are used close to your body. Radio frequency sources such as computer video monitors, radio and TV broadcast transmitters, amateur (ham) radios, cellular telephones, and other communication devices also emit EM waves. See the graph *Typical electric and magnetic fields near equipment* for further information.

As these devices proliferate, scientists and the public increasingly are asking whether exposure to EM fields involves risk to human health. A lot of sound scientific research has been done, but the answers still remain unclear. There are indications that prolonged exposure to EM radiation can cause health problems including cancer. Several recent epidemiologic studies indicate that there may be health dangers from repeated exposure to a specific frequency, 50 or 60 Hertz (Hz), used for electrical power transmission throughout the world. On the other hand a large number of other studies have found no increased health risks associated with EM fields.

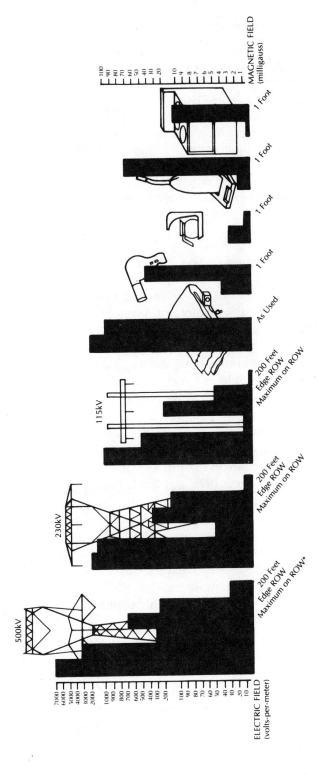

E/MF get smaller as you move away from equipment. Beyond 3 to 5 feet, appliance magnetic fields are less than 1 milligauss, and electric fields are less than 10 volts-per-meter. There is no **magnetic** field around an appliance when it is turned off. There is an **electric** field whenever equipment is plugged in.

*Right of Way

Typical electric and magnetic fields near equipment. (*Source: Electric Power Lines: Q&A on Research into Health Effects*, Bonneville Power Administration, Portland, Oregon.)

The Electrical Current Used to Power Our Homes

The electric power we use in our homes, offices, and factories is alternating current (AC). This is in contrast to the direct current (DC) that is produced by batteries. An alternating current doesn't flow steadily in one direction; it alternates back and forth. The power we use in North America alternates back and forth 60 times each second. Scientists call this 60 Hz power. In Europe and some other parts of the world the frequency of electric power is 50 Hz rather than 60 Hz.

Possible Dangers from EM Radiation

The concern is that prolonged exposure to EM fields at 50/60 Hz frequencies might increase one's chances of developing cancer. This concern is prompted by evidence from epidemiologic studies of children. Four of seven cases of children with cancer of the nervous system, leukemia, and/or lymphomas have shown that those who live in houses located near 60 Hz electric transmission and distribution lines have "modestly elevated risks" of developing cancer compared to control groups.

One of the most frequently cited studies was done by Dr. David Savitz, while professor at the University of Colorado Medical School. He did a case-control analysis of 356 childhood cancer cases in the Denver area between 1976 and 1983. From this study he calculated a risk ratio of 1.5; that is, children with cancer were about $1\frac{1}{2}$ times more likely to live near high voltage–carrying power lines than were children who did not develop cancer.

Epidemiological case studies such as these are often considered problematic because they are prey to what scientists call "confounding factors"—factors other than those studied that may cause the "discovered effect" (in this case, cancer). This problem caused one top researcher to focus on just that: He studied potential confounders and biases, looking for factors that might have affected the results in these studies. However, he concluded that "no other agents have been identified that could explain" the association between EM fields and cancer. Other scientists, however, are not convinced that all other possible confounding factors have been eliminated.

So, even though there are questions about the design of these studies, their combined results are sobering. They serve as a warning of a possible health danger. But how much danger is there and what should be done about it? At this early date, experts just don't know because of insufficient data. Studies are continuing, and there may be clearer answers in the near future.

Ever since the pioneering discoveries of Pierre and Marie Curie (Marie died of sickness caused by repeated exposure to radium, one of the two radioactive elements she discovered) we have known that too much exposure to ionizing radiation can cause cancer. Ionizing radiation produces rays and/or particles energetic enough to dislodge electrons from the atoms or molecules they encounter in our bodies. However, EM fields produce non-ionizing radiation—radiation too weak to dislodge electrons. Although certain forms of non-ionizing radiation such as ultraviolet light and microwaves can have an adverse effect on living organisms (microwaves will be discussed later in this chapter), EM radiation was generally thought to be safe. This long-held belief is now being seriously questioned. According to the EPA: "We lack key information necessary to make a judgment as to how far one should live from high-power transmission lines to be safe. We don't know how risky it is to actually live under such transmission lines."

If authorities don't know much about the EM risk from high-voltage transmission lines, what about risks from low-voltage electrical appliance sources such as microwave ovens?

Microwave Radiation

More than 80 percent of U.S. households have one or more microwave ovens. Microwave ovens produce EM energy that heats the water molecules in food but passes through glass, paper, and plastic. This EM energy can also pass through our bodies. Does that ability make microwave ovens dangerous? Not unless you climb into your microwave oven. These ovens are designed with shielding to prevent leakage of harmful levels of microwave energy. Even if a broken microwave leaks radiation, distance away from the source of microwave energy provides protection. It doesn't have to be a lot of distance—one to three feet of space away from a source of microwave radiation provides adequate protection.

It's important to put the possibility of microwave danger into context. We are all continuously bombarded with microwaves from such diverse sources as military and civilian radar installations, radio and television transmitters, communications and surveillance satellites, transmitters at airports and on planes and ships, telephone and TV signal relay towers, walkie-talkies, video display terminals, and automatic garage door openers, as well as microwave ovens. Whether or not the *cumulative effect* of microwave radiation presents a health threat remains a matter of controversy among researchers.

How to Protect Your Family

Some experts and members of the public have concluded that since knowledge about the possible health effects of EM fields is so scanty no action is justified at this stage. Others feel that something should be done because the evidence does point to some risk.

Ambiguities and unanswered questions allow few solid answers about what to do, but most authorities do agree that *frequency of exposure and nearness to EM transmission sources are important determinants of risk*. The strength of an EM field diminishes rapidly as you move away from the source just as the light from a candle, or the heat from a campfire, diminishes as you move away from it. That knowledge leads us to one possible line of action: *prudent avoidance,* a term coined by Granger Morton, a professor in the department of Electrical and Computer Engineering at Carnegie-Mellon University. If you want to reduce your EM exposure, practice prudent avoidance.

First, start by looking for small electric motors that you or members of your family are often close to. You might have an electric blanket bombarding you with EM fields throughout the night, or you might be close to a computer's video monitor for most of the day. Another possible EM source in your home is the motor-driven electric clock on your bedside table. It can produce a fairly strong magnetic field by your head. Practice prudent avoidance by moving it to a dresser across the room, or replace it with a battery-driven or wind-up clock.

Second, learn to turn off appliances not being used. Current does not have to be flowing for an *electrical* field to exist. That explains why it's possible to get an electric shock from an appliance that is plugged in, but turned off. The appliance doesn't produce a *magnetic* field until it is turned on and electrical current flows. The flowing electricity produces a magnetic field; stronger currents produce stronger fields. For example, the EM field generated by a hair

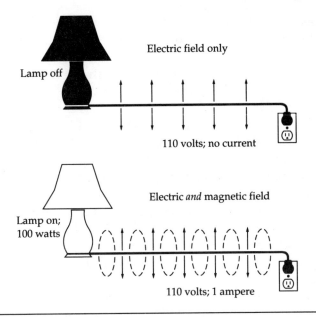

Lamp off

Electric field only

110 volts; no current

Lamp on;
100 watts

Electric *and* magnetic field

110 volts; 1 ampere

Electric versus electromagnetic fields. (*Source:* Bonneville Power Administration, Portland, Oregon.)

dryer will be higher when the dryer is operated on its "high heat" setting (when it draws a lot of current) than when it is operated on its "low heat" setting. See the drawing of the lamps *Electric versus electromagnetic fields.*

Third, since distance from the appliance is important, don't be closer than necessary to appliances when they are in use. For instance, the strength of a microwave oven's EM field is 10 to 20 times weaker a foot away from the oven than it is an inch away from the oven. If you move three feet away, the strength of the field is about 100 times weaker.

Use the same common-sense distancing safety measures with other electrical appliances. For instance, since an electric blanket lies directly on the body for hours at a time, it's best not to use it throughout the night. (Studies have shown that children whose mothers had used electric blankets during the first trimester of pregnancy were 30 percent more likely to develop cancer.) It is safe to use an electric blanket to warm your bed if you unplug it before going to bed. Better yet, use a heavy quilt and cuddle up to your favorite warm-blooded person.

**TROUBLESHOOTING GUIDE TO REDUCING YOUR FAMILY'S EM RADI-
ATION EXPOSURE**   Here is more prudent avoidance advice:

Air conditioners. Don't sit closer than three feet away for long
periods, even with just the fan on.

Bedside appliances. Electric clocks and fans usually run continuously. They should be kept at least 30 inches from the head.

Cellular and portable phones, CB radios. These are used close to the
head and body so there might be some risk. However, since they
are usually used for short durations, the risk is probably very low.
Recommendation: Don't use unnecessarily.

Electric baseboard and space heaters. Since these are in use for long
periods of time, take precautions by placing beds, especially children's, at least three feet away. Don't place beds or cribs on the
other side of walls that heaters are up against because magnetic fields
penetrate walls.

Electric shavers and hair dryers. These produce strong EM fields,
but exposure is of short duration so risk is minimal.

Electric water bed heaters. Heat the water in the water bed before
going to bed, then turn off the heater. If the water in your bed cools
too quickly to be comfortable during the night, consider hooking
the heater to a timer to start the heater for a minimum amount of
time during the night.

Fluorescent lights. For desk lamps, it's better to switch to incan-
descent bulbs. Fluorescent ceiling fixtures are probably safe because
they're far enough away from the body.

Microwave ovens. Some experts advise that you have a service person check the door gasket annually for microwave radiation leakage,
and stand a few feet away while the microwave is on.

Refrigerators, washers, and dryers. These appliances produce strong
EM fields when they are running (for refrigerators, that means almost constantly). EM fields are concentrated at the back of these
machines, so don't place beds or cribs on the other side of walls
they're up against.

Audio systems, laser computer printers, or copiers. Place at least three
feet away from your seating area.

Video monitors and TVs. These generate EM fields in all directions, not just from their screens. Sit at least an arm's distance
or three feet away from video monitors. For safety, sit at least six
feet away from 19-inch TVs and eight feet from larger ones. Turn off

video monitors and televisions when not in use. Don't place cribs or beds on the other side of walls where televisions or video monitors are located.

Points to Remember When Considering a Move

If you are considering a move to a new home, consider the location and distribution of electric power lines. Try to avoid being close to high-voltage transmission wires or electric-generating substations. Make sure that the main electrical line connecting your house to the outside electrical network doesn't enter your home within several feet of bedrooms or anywhere else members of your family spend a lot of time.

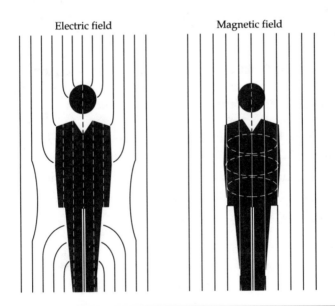

Electric and magnetic fields passing through a person. Electric and magnetic fields from electrical appliances and from power lines induce weak electrical currents in people and animals. Solid lines represent invisible fields. Dotted lines indicate the direction of induced current flow. This drawing shows a person standing directly under a power line. (*Source:* Bonneville Power Administration, Portland, Oregon.)

Quick Summary

Electric and magnetic fields are found wherever there is electric power. This means that electromagnetic fields are found around all electrical transmission and distribution lines, all home wiring, and all electrical appliances.

Some studies indicate that prolonged exposure to EM fields can cause health problems, including cancer. Don't panic. The studies are cause for concern; however, the evidence they provide is far from conclusive. Studies are continuing. Some experts, including the authors of this book, believe it may be wise to practice *prudent avoidance*. That means reducing one's exposure to EM fields by turning off electrical appliances not being used and putting a reasonable amount of distance between yourself and EM-emitting objects.

Remember, even if EM fields are ultimately demonstrated to pose a health risk, keep the danger they present in perspective. Other factors such as street traffic and crime patterns, as well as radon levels or lead poisoning in your dwelling are likely to be even more significant in terms of your own and your children's overall safety.

ADDITIONAL RESOURCES The Bonneville Power Administration, a federal agency, has three free publications on the biological effects and possible health hazards of EM fields. They are:

- Electric and Magnetic Fields from 60–Hertz Electric Power: What Do We Know About Possible Health Risks?
- Electrical and Biological Effects of Transmission Lines: A Review.
- Electric Power Lines: Questions and Answers on Research into Health Effects.

Write Bonneville Power Administration, P.O. Box 12999, Portland OR 97212; or call toll-free: 800-547-6048.

CHAPTER 12

HAZARDOUS NOISE

Sound Advice

Our world is a noisy place. According to the EPA, nearly half of all Americans are regularly exposed to levels of noise that interfere with important natural activities such as speaking, listening, sleeping, or working. Several years ago a Gallup poll taken among city dwellers revealed that most consider excessive noise as second only to water pollution among environmental issues of concern to them. In fact, the respondents to the survey, which ranked the qualities of an ideal neighborhood, said quiet surroundings were as important as low crime rates, friendly people, and good housing. Quiet was considered *more* important than good schools, low traffic volume, and easily accessible shopping areas. Another study, by the U.S. Department of Housing and Urban Development, found that city residents most often named noise as the worst characteristic of their neighborhoods. Noise and crime were cited as the two major factors that caused people to wish that they could move to another part of town.

Health Effects of
Excessive Noise Levels

Until recently, most people considered noise simply a nuisance, but we now know that noise can be hazardous to our health. The National Institute on Deafness and Other Communication Disorders (NIDCD) states that it is generally accepted by medical experts that sustained sound levels over 85 decibels—sounds roughly equivalent to those produced by a food blender, power lawn mower, or power leaf blower—are potentially dangerous and can lead to noise-induced hearing loss and possibly other health problems.

> Calling noise a nuisance is like calling smog an inconvenience. Noise must be considered a hazard to the health of people everywhere.
>
> *William H. Steward, former U.S. Surgeon General.*

Hearing loss afflicts nearly 30 million Americans, according to an NIDCD Consensus Development Conference. Approximately one-third, almost 10 million of these people, suffered impairment at least partially attributable to damage from exposure to loud sounds. And sounds that are loud enough to damage sensitive inner ear structures can produce hearing loss that is not reversible by any currently available medical or surgical treatment.

Perhaps even more alarming than the threat of hearing loss is recent research showing that noise can affect blood pressure, body chemistry, ability to sleep, and even our ability to acquire knowledge! There is even evidence that noise suppresses the immune system, thereby impairing our resistance to disease. In addition, UCLA scientists found a high rate of death from heart attacks, strokes, suicides, and murder among 200,000 residents of a noisy flight-path corridor near Los Angeles International Airport compared to the rest of the city.

Studies have shown that noisy surroundings in the home and at school can adversely affect children's ability to learn, specifically impeding their language development and their ability to read. Gifted children—described as those with IQ levels above 130–140 and those of artistic inclination—are especially at risk. Studies indicate they are more aware of noise and are more disturbed by it than children of average intelligence.

Children may be at particular risk because the dimensions and configuration of their auditory canals are different than those of adults. Research indicates that this difference may make youngsters more likely to sustain trauma to the tympanic membrane and middle ear. However, hearing impairment associated with noise exposure can occur at any age.

It is also known that noise can penetrate the womb and provoke responses in the developing unborn child. Research reveals that a fetus responds to loud noise with increased heart rate and kicking. A Japanese study suggests that expectant mothers living in noisy environments are more likely to give birth to underweight babies than are women from quieter areas.

WARNING SIGNS OF NOISE–INDUCED HEARING LOSS Because hearing loss is gradual and because the inner ear has no mechanism for registering pain, it is difficult to persuade some people that their hearing is fading or at risk from harmful noise levels. Nevertheless, there are certain signs that warn of permanent hearing damage. If heeded early enough, these warnings can help prevent more serious damage. The warning signs are:

- Inability to hear high-pitched or soft sounds
- Trouble understanding phone conversations
- Difficulty in conducting conversations when there are high levels of background noise (when one is experiencing hearing loss, high levels of background noise tend to block out conversational sounds that people with normal hearing can understand)
- Sensations of unsteadiness, dizziness, or nausea during noise exposure
- Great tension and irritability after prolonged noise exposure
- Hearing a ringing or roaring sound in the ears for several hours after being exposed to loud sounds

Unfortunately, the only dependable way to determine if you are suffering noise-induced hearing loss is to have a hearing test by a physician or an audiologist. One way to find out if you should consider such an exam is to take a simple telephone screening test. Call 800-222-EARS between 9 A.M. and 6 P.M. Eastern time to reach a national operator who will give you a phone number in your region. (Exceptions: In Pennsylvania, call 800-345-EARS; in Canada, 215-359-1144. The 800 number is free, but the regional number may be long distance and would be charged to you at standard rates.) When you call, you'll reach an answering machine that will tell you to listen for four faint tones in each ear. Thus it's important to call from a quiet area, away from sounds made by voices, TV, air conditioners, or traffic. If you can't hear some or all of the tones, don't panic. It may have something to do with the phone you are using. And even normal ears vary in their sensitivity from day to day. Wait a few days and call again using another phone. If you get the same results, you should consider getting a hearing test. Even if you hear all the tones, but show some of the other signs of hearing problems, see a doctor.

Our Homes Are No Longer a Haven from Noise

The unit of measurement used to monitor the amplitude, or intensity, of sound is called a decibel (dB). As shown earlier in this chapter, the more intense a sound, the higher the dB level, and permanent hearing loss is generally associated with noise levels in excess of 85 dB. The table *Common noise levels around the house* gives amplitude levels measured in decibels for some common home and garden appliances and tools.

Compare the sound levels of common household appliances in the first table with the next table, *Sound levels and human response,* developed by the EPA. You'll see that many appliances and tools

Common Noise Levels Around the House

Noise Source	Sound Level in Decibels
Refrigerator	40
Floor fan	38 to 70
Clothes dryer	55
Washing machine	47 to 78
Dishwasher	54 to 85
Hair dryer	59 to 80
Vacuum cleaner	62 to 85
Sewing machine	64 to 74
Electric shaver	75
Sink garbage disposal	67 to 93
Alarm clock	80
Electric lawn edger	81
Home shop tools	85
Gasoline power mower	87 to 92
Gasoline riding mower	90 to 95
Gasoline-powered leaf blower	100
Chain saw	100
Stereo	Up to 120

produce sound that is considered intrusive, annoying, or even dangerous to human hearing.

At one time or another almost everyone has experienced annoyance or irritation due to noise, but most of us have been unaware that the sounds that produce annoyance may also be permanently affecting our hearing. Most people are familiar with the feeling of temporary deafness and ringing in the ears that can follow sudden exposure to a very loud noise, such as a firecracker exploding nearby. This type of partial hearing loss, called temporary threshold shift (TTS), usually lasts only a few hours at most. However, only recently has it been recognized that regular exposure to noise levels commonly encountered in everyday life (such as city traffic) can, over a period of time, result in permanent hearing loss. Because damage to hearing is usually painless, few people recognize that the injury is occurring until it is too late. Although for most people permanent hearing loss can occur when daily noise levels are about 85 dB or more, for particularly sensitive individuals average sound levels as low as 70 dB may be dangerous.

Household appliances and tools including dishwashers, hair dryers, vacuum cleaners, food processors, mowers, lawn edgers, hedge trimmers, and chain saws can all generate sound levels that

Sound Levels and Human Response

Common Sounds	Noise Level (dB)	Effect
Air raid siren	140	Danger zone for hearing damage
Jet takeoff	130	
Discotheque	120	
Pile driver	110	
Garbage truck	100	
City traffic	90	Very annoying, hearing damage
Alarm clock	80	Annoying
Freeway traffic	70	Phone use difficult
Air-conditioning	60	Intrusive
Light auto traffic	50	Quiet
Living room	40	
Library	30	Very quiet
Broadcasting studio	20	
A whisper	10	Just audible

can interrupt conversations, be disturbing to neighbors, or even result in permanent damage to the ears. Alone or used briefly, they only irritate and annoy, but prolonged use and the cumulative decibel levels of several household appliances (plus the background din of a TV or a radio) can add together to produce dangerous noise pollution in our homes.

Because the decibel scale is a logarithmic measure of sound intensity, decibel values don't add up in the usual way. A 10 dB difference means one sound is 10 times louder than another. A New York subway is about 100 decibels, but a boom box or live rock band blasting at 110 dB is a bone-jarring ten times louder. Customized car stereos that boast several speakers can blare their music at 120 to 130 dB—that's 100 to 1,000 times louder than a New York subway and roughly equivalent to the sound of a jet engine at takeoff. At these intensities, even a small increase or reduction in decibel values can make a significant difference in noise intensity.

How to Protect Your Family

There are three ways to control sound transmission in the home:

1. By increasing the thickness of the walls, floors, or ceilings
2. By breaking the path of vibration through the air
3. By a method called *cavity absorption*

If you are thinking of buying or building a new home, knowing about these three methods may help you make decisions that will result in a quieter home.

In your present home it's probably impractical to think of increasing the thickness of the structure's walls; nevertheless you can break the path of sound vibration by hanging rugs or tapestries on the wall or by simply closing doors between noise-prone areas, such as the kitchen or laundry room, and living areas. If the doors currently installed don't do a good job of dampening the sound, they are probably not solid-core or insulated doors. You may consider installing better doors. Breaking the path of sound vibration can reduce sound intensity by as much as 6 to 10 decibels.

Cavity absorption involves the use of mineral fiber insulation to fill the spaces in walls, floors, and ceilings. This type of renovation can further decrease sound levels by 5 to 15 decibels, according to the Mineral Insulation Manufacturers Association.

Here are some other practical and efficient steps that you can take to reduce sound levels in your home:

- Set rules for your children regarding the sound intensity at which the TV, radio, or stereo may be played. Instruct them in why it is important *not* to play sound equipment at full intensity.
- When you use tools in the workshop or use the lawn mower or other noisy machinery, wear earplugs to protect your hearing.
- Warn children about the dangers of playing with loud toys, such as cap guns, close to anyone's ears, or don't purchase such toys in the first place.
- When purchasing new appliances, select quiet ones. When evaluating appliances, be aware that because of loud background noise levels in most stores, an appliance can sound louder at home than in the store.
- When purchasing air-conditioning or ventilation equipment, make sure they have quiet motors and well-balanced fans that do not give off sound-producing vibrations.
- Locate heating and cooling equipment far from bedrooms. If that's not possible, consider insulating them by building a small enclosure around them or by walling them off.
- Mount equipment, such as window air conditioners, firmly so as to keep vibration to a minimum.
- To further soundproof your home, consider caulking all unnecessary openings in walls and floors.
- In noisy areas, consider installing acoustical tile ceilings.
- Turn down the ringers on your phones to reduce sound intensity.
- Consider purchasing a noise suppresser. "White sound" or sleep sound generators are small electrical units that produce a soft whooshing, the sound of rainfall, or pounding surf. They often successfully muffle or camouflage sounds such as rattling radiators, traffic noise, conversations, or even snoring. These table-top machines cost from $50 to $150.

Quick Summary

Too often our homes aren't safe havens from noise. Noise levels may increase because of appliances we've purchased to make our lives easier or because of the improper use of home entertainment equipment. Dishwashers, hair dryers, air-conditioning systems, garbage disposals, lawn mowers, and TV and stereo equipment all contribute to high sound levels that collectively may cause adverse health effects including damage to our hearing. If you are buying or building a new home or if you are already established in a home, there are steps you can take to create a safe, quiet environment.

ADDITIONAL RESOURCES   If you suspect you need help for hearing loss, contact the American Speech-Language-Hearing Association (ASHA) at 800-638-8255; or, in Maryland, Alaska, and Hawaii, 301-897-8682. Or write ASHA at: 10801 Rockville Pike, Rockville MD 20852.

If you are planning to build a new home, the Mineral Insulation Manufacturers Association (MIMA) has a free booklet that explains recommended construction methods for controlling sounds. Write: MIMA, 1420 King St, Alexandria VA 22314, for *Sound Control for Commercial and Residential Buildings*. Other free booklets that offer similar advice include:

- *Fire Resistance and Sound Control Guide,* from CertainTeed Corp., P.O. Box 860, Valley Forge PA 19482.

- *Sound Control,* from Manville Building Materials Corp., Ken-Caryl Ranch, Denver CO 80217.

- *Noise Control Design in Residential Construction,* from Owens-Corning Fiberglas, Insulation Operating Division, Fiberglas Tower, Toledo OH 43659.

CHAPTER 13

"AN OUNCE OF PREVENTION"

Healthy Cocooning

"An ounce of prevention is worth a pound of cure" whether you are building a home, buying an older home, or maintaining the one you currently own.

Creating a healthy, safe, comfortable, and secure home depends on the decisions you make and the actions you take *before* you buy or build a house as well as the decisions and purchases you make while living there. These decisions include limiting sources of indoor air pollutants by using nontoxic building materials. After you move in, these good decisions continue when you buy environmentally safe consumer products to use within the home.

A healthy and safe home is one that is designed and built to ensure that its inhabitants breathe clean air and drink clean water. It provides a safe haven from the dangers of air and water pollution, lead, radon, pesticides, and carbon monoxide. A healthy and safe home is designed and constructed to reduce the chances of allergic reactions and asthma attacks caused by pollens, dusts, and molds. It is designed and built so as not to be a major source of indoor pollutants such as asbestos, chemical fumes, combustion products, and microbiological organisms that can cause breathing and other health difficulties.

Factors to Consider When Building a New Home

When building a new home, there are at least two levels of protection that can be built into the home. The first level, a minimum protective level, should include the following:

- A dry basement, with no mold or mildew problems
- No elevated radon levels
- No asbestos materials used in the home
- No lead in the plumbing
- Lowest-risk pesticides, if needed, applied carefully
- Kitchen and bathroom exhaust fans

Beyond this minimum level and because of the potential for significantly improving the indoor environment, consumers building their own homes may want to consider, if they can afford them, the following options:

- Whole-house ventilation system, with or without a heat recovery system
- Filtration systems for air and water
- Central vacuum system that exhausts house dust outside
- No building materials made with formaldehyde such as formaldehyde-containing particleboard, paneling, cabinets, carpets, carpet pads, carpet adhesives, paints, or finishes.

Although many different toxic chemicals are contained in building materials, most outgas in a relatively short interval after construction. Formaldehyde, however, can give off fumes for years. Thus it is especially important to avoid products that contain high amounts of formaldehyde such as urea-formaldehyde foam insulation, particleboard, chipboard, waferboard, composition board, and medium-density fiberboard. These products are commonly used in countertops, kitchen and bathroom cabinets, floor underlayment, roof and wall sheathing, shelving, and furniture.

As alternatives, use solid wood or exterior grade plywood, which uses the less harmful form of formaldehyde, phenol-formaldehyde. Most oriented-strandboard (OSB) uses phenol-formaldehyde. If you must use formaldehyde-containing products, prevent or reduce outgasing by sealing the products with alkyl-based paint or polyurethane.

Remember, the first line of defense against indoor air pollution is to reduce or eliminate the source of pollutants. For that reason, have your builder mix all paints and finishes outside the home whenever possible to keep fumes from saturating the home. Make sure the builder ventilates the home while applying these products and continues to ventilate the home until all volatile solvents have evaporated and no odor is detected.

Here's a chart of factors to consider when building your new home.

Potential Construction Problems and Solutions

Problem	Pollutant Danger	Solution
Water runoff can collect, causing wet basement	Can result in mold growth, causing allergic reactions	Build on well-drained land; choose high ground with a low water table
Water pollution from groundwater, central system, or wells	Organic and inorganic chemicals and microorganisms including lead	Test and filter water
Radon gas in soil	Radon decay products increase lung cancer risk	Purchase land elsewhere; or if radon levels can be handled, seal slab, put 4 inches of gravel under slab; use sub-slab ventilation
Pesticide-drenched soil	Pesticide poisoning and resulting health difficulties	Test soil and avoid a contaminated site
Highway pollution	Noise, lead, smog, dust, carbon dioxide, and carbon monoxide	Locate homes away from busy streets or plant a buffer area of trees and shrubs
Hazardous waste site	Numerous toxic wastes can cause a variety of health difficulties	Investigate before purchasing site; build elsewhere
Trash in backfill	May attract termites and require pesticides	Use termite shields, clean backfill, apply nontoxic pesticides

(Continued)

Potential Construction Problems and Solutions *(Continued)*

Problem	Pollutant Danger	Solution
Formaldehyde in building materials	Respiratory distress	Avoid. Use exterior-grade plywood or low formaldehyde-emitting boards with alkyl-based paint or polyurethane
Asbestos tiles or shingles	Abestos causes lung cancer	Avoid using and never cut or sand
Backdrafting of combustion products	Various combustion products cause a variety of ills	Use sealed combustion, electric appliances, or forced vent systems
Excess humidity from bathrooms and laundry rooms	Provides breeding material for mold, mildew, and biological contaminants	Install exhaust fans
Suspended respirable particulates such as dust and tobacco smoke	Allergies from dust, mold, pollen, and other airborne particles	Install high-efficiency air filtration system; install central vacuum cleaner with outside exhaust; don't smoke.
Lead from water pipes and solder in plumbing	Lead can impair the neurological system	Use plastic pipe or lead-free solder

Buying an Older Home

Many of the factors that one considers if building a home should be reviewed by a person deciding to purchase an existing house. For instance, does the house have a damp basement? Is there excess humidity in bathrooms and laundry rooms? If the house is musty, there might be a potential problem with allergies from mold. Only you can decide if the potential problems can be dealt with and if the advantages of the house outweigh the disadvantages of needing to fix potential difficulties.

There are many other problems unique to older homes—problems such as lead plumbing, or lead solder on pipes, and asbestos in tiles and shingles. Are you willing to bear the expense and hassle of lead or asbestos mitigation projects? Also, have you tested for radon?

Maintaining Your Home for Health and Safety

To make sure your home stays healthy, you have to continue to take steps to keep it that way. Remember the three basic strategies to improve air quality in the home: In reverse order of importance they include air cleaning, improving ventilation, and preventing sources of pollutants from ever coming in. We've talked about all three strategies before, but let's review a few source-control tips that bear emphasizing.

- If you smoke, stop! Discourage smoking by others in your home. As we have explained, scientific evidence indicates that secondary smoke increases the risks of lung cancer, heart attack, and health difficulties. Combined with radon or asbestos exposure, tobacco smoke becomes even deadlier.

- Use the bathroom exhaust fan or open the window at least a few inches while showering. This significantly reduces exposure to chloroform generated when the hot chlorinated water of the shower hits surface areas.

- Avoid the use of room deodorizers and other aerosol products such as hairsprays. Avoiding such products will substantially reduce the air pollutant burden found in most homes since hairspray aerosols are the number one producer of household hydrocarbons followed by window washing sprays and room air freshener sprays.

- Use nontoxic alternatives to pesticides whenever possible.

- Air out dry-cleaned clothes on a balcony or a porch for a day. According to the EPA, "garments recently dry-cleaned are the major source of personal exposure to tetrachloroethylene," the solvent of choice for dry-cleaning. This chemical has been shown to cause cancer in animals.

Room-by-Room
Health and Safety Tips

Here's a final room-by-room health checklist that can help you provide a healthy and safe house to protect your family over the long term.

- Your fireplace or wood stove should be properly vented to the outside. Have the chimney cleaned yearly. Be careful never to burn green, wet, painted or treated wood, trash or garbage, plastics, magazines, colored paper, or gift wrap. These materials can give off harmful chemicals such as lead that can pollute your indoor air.

- If you have new wall-to-wall carpet, increase ventilation for 48 hours after installation. Don't drench with pesticides or chemical preservatives or antistain coatings. Many people consider area rugs to be better than wall-to-wall carpeting because they can be picked up and washed in hot water of at least 130°F, to reduce dust mites.

- If you have drapes or paneling that may still be emitting formaldehyde gas, increase ventilation.

- Periodically check wiring, and replace frayed or cracked electrical wiring in all rooms.

- Remove peeling paint, but first have it tested to determine if it is lead or mercury-based. If it is, hire professionals experienced in the safe removal of lead or mercury paint.

- If you have acoustic ceiling tile that begins to crumble, have it tested for asbestos and if it is, hire professionals to remove. Cover exposed asbestos with plastic or duct tape for an air-tight seal. Never try to remove it yourself because the fibers will only become airborne, increasing the risk of contamination.

- Keep your entire house clean to reduce exposure to house dust mites, pollens, animal dander, and other allergy-causing agents. (Have people who are allergic to these agents leave the house while vacuuming because it can increase levels of airborne mite allergens.) Frequent cleaning of smooth surfaces with a wet cloth or mop can also reduce the amount of dust and other particulates in the home.

- If you have small children, make sure that toxic cleaning products are out-of-sight and secured with safety latches. Read the small print on all household product containers and follow directions carefully.

- Fit your gas range with a hood that vents pollutants outdoors. If the tips of your gas range flames are yellow or orange instead of blue, adjust the range. Never use your gas stove to heat your home.

- Do not use old or imported dishes or pottery that may contain lead in the glaze or paint. If you forget and do use antique glass that may be lead-glazed or painted, do not wash in the dishwasher because the hot water and detergent can loosen the lead.

- Refrigerator drip pans should be emptied and cleaned regularly.

- If carpets or other materials become water-logged, thoroughly dry and clean them within 24 hours if possible to prevent the growth of mold and bacteria. If health problems occur and persist after you have tried to dry these materials, you may have to totally replace them because it is very difficult to completely rid such materials of biological contaminants.

- Paradichlorobenzene, which causes cancer in animals, is a constituent of mothproofing products and air deodorizers. Consider using natural repellents such as cedar chips, dried lavender, or pennyroyal leaves.

- If you or members of your family have allergies, use synthetic or foam rubber mattress pads and pillows. Wash them frequently. Avoid fuzzy wool blankets, feather or wool-stuffed comforters, and feather pillows.

- Do not allow film and scale to develop in your humidifier or dehumidifier. Use distilled or demineralized water to reduce the building of mineral scale. Clean humidifiers and dehumidifiers frequently. Use a brush or other scrubber to clean the tank. If you use chlorine bleach or other cleaning products or disinfectants, make sure you rinse the tank well to avoid breathing harmful chemicals.

- Fix any water seepage into the basement. Fix any leaky pipes to tubs and sinks. Put a plastic cover over dirt in crawl spaces to prevent moisture from rising from the ground and entering the house. Be sure crawl spaces are well ventilated. Pay special attention to carpet on concrete floors because carpets absorb moisture readily. If you plan to install a wall-to-wall carpet in a basement recreation room, it may be necessary to use a vapor barrier composed of plastic sheeting over the concrete. Cover the plastic sheeting with exterior-grade plywood, then install the carpeting.

- If you use toxic materials in a hobby—such as paint thinner, turpentine, or pottery glazes—vacuum or damp-mop the hobby rooms frequently in order to pick up toxic substances before they dry up, become airborne, and are inhaled.

- Workers at poison control centers testify to how often children swallow turpentine, pesticides, or other toxic substances. It is extremely important to keep such substances out of the reach of small children and to lock up the hobby room, workshop, and garage to keep small children out.

- Read all the print on containers and follow directions carefully when using household cleaning agents, hobby materials, and pesticides. Where feasible, substitute pump-type products for aerosols.

- To prevent the buildup of carbon monoxide (a silent, odorless killer) never leave a car or lawnmower engine running in the garage or any enclosed space.

- Have your gas or oil company annually inspect your furnace, gas water heater, and gas clothes dryers for potential leaks.

- Clean and disinfect the basement floor drain regularly. It can be a hotspot of biological pollutants that could spread throughout the home.

- If there is too much dampness in your home, operate a dehumidifier in the basement or, if necessary, in other areas of the house.

- Remove chemical substances from your workshop and garage when you no longer need them.

The Trend toward Cocooning

People are increasingly *cocooning*—staying put to enjoy their homes as sanctuaries from the hustle and stress of the workplace. According to a Gallup poll commissioned by *Newsweek* magazine, 70 percent of the adults surveyed said that staying at home is their favorite way to spend an evening.

Since the majority of us are staying home more, it makes sense to make our homes as safe, healthy, and convenient as possible. You now know what needs to be done to help ensure your health and safety and the health and safety of your loved ones. Whether you are building a new home, buying an older home, or maintaining an established home, you can prevent many of the problems that make up the "sick house" syndrome and result in needless illness. Have a healthy home and a healthier family. Good luck. May your home be your haven, may your family enjoy good health, safety, comfort, and the time you need to enjoy it all.

APPENDIX

Resource Directories

When one has a home health problem, the question of whom to call for advice and information is often a source of frustration. There are hundreds of public agencies and private firms that might help. These directories of state, federal, and private organizations are powerful tools that will help you cut straight through the clutter of different agencies to find the help you need. The directories are a guide to locating people who can provide you with information and assistance on home health and safety problems. The directories bring together public contact listings on 18 topics, from asbestos to water pollution, in the health departments and other public agencies of the 50 state governments as well as the federal government. Also included are EPA regional offices, hotline information sources, and private organizations.

The information in Directory A is organized alphabetically by state. For each state, the directory lists the various types of home health problems, followed by a listing of agencies within the state that deal with such problems. Where possible, individuals to contact are named. Addresses and telephone numbers are included.

In general, the contacts listed are able to provide useful information and appropriate referrals. However, programs and resources devoted to home health and safety issues vary widely from state to state. For instance, you may want to call to find out if your home can be inspected for potential indoor air quality or water pollution problems. Some state and local agencies conduct on-site home inspections; many do not. Telephone consultation with state or local personnel will, at best, result in direct aid to answer your questions and find solutions or, at least, put you in contact with officials who can make referrals to commercial firms to help you solve your problem.

Directory A
State Contacts for Healthy Home Issues

ALABAMA

Asbestos, Formaldehyde, Home Health Complaints, Radon, and Other Indoor Air Pollutants

Indoor Air Quality Branch
(for radon, Division of Radiation Control)
Alabama Department of Public Health
434 Monroe St
Montgomery AL 36130
205-242-5095

Pesticides, Termiticides, and Chlordane

John A. Bloch
Alabama Department of Agriculture and Industry
Agriculture Chemistry/Plant Industry Division
P.O. Box 3336
Montgomery AL 36193
205-242-2656

ALASKA

Asbestos, Biologicals, Home Health Complaints

Alaska Department of Health and Social Services
Division of Public Health, Box H
Juneau AK 99811-0613
907-465-3019

Pesticides, Termiticides, Chlordane, Wood Preservatives

William Burgoyne, Ph.D.
Alaska Department of Environmental Conservation
Division of Environmental Health
P.O. Box O
Juneau AK 99811-1800
907-273-9448

ARIZONA

Asbestos, Biologicals, Combustion Devices and Gases, Formaldehyde, Insulation, Paints, Solvents and Cleaners, Home-Related Health Complaints

Norm Peterson
Office of Risk Assessment
Arizona Department of Health Services
3008 N Third St
Phoenix AZ 85012
602-257-5857

Particulates

James Guyton
Arizona Department of Environmental Quality
Office of Air Quality
2005 N Central Ave
Phoenix AZ 85004
602-257-2339

Pesticides

Jack Root
Arizona Structural Pest Control Commission
1150 S Priest #4
Tempe AZ 85281

Radon

Paul Weeden
Arizona Radiation Regulatory Agency
4814 S 40th St
Phoenix AZ 85040
602-255-4845

ARKANSAS

*Asbestos, Biologicals, Combustion Devices and Gases,
Formaldehyde, Insulation, Lead (in paint), Paints, Solvents
and Cleaners, Particulates, Pesticides, Radon*

Arkansas Department of Health
Bureau of Environmental Health Services
4815 W Markham St
Little Rock AR 72205
501-661-2000

CALIFORNIA

Asbestos, Biologicals, Combustion Devices and Gases, Formaldehyde, Insulation, Lead (in paint), Paints, Solvents and Cleaners, Particulates, Pesticides, Radon

California Department of Health Services
2151 Berkeley Way
Berkeley CA 94704
415-540-3324

Also for Formaldehyde and Insulation Information:
Gordon Damant
California Department of Consumer Affairs
Bureau of Home Furnishings and Thermal Insulation
3485 Orange Grove Avenue
North Highlands CA 95660
916-920-6951

Also for Pesticide Information:
Rex Mages, Division of Pest Management
California Department of Food and Agriculture
1220 N. Street
Sacramento CA 95814
916-654-0551

COLORADO

Asbestos, Biologicals, Combustion Devices and Gases, Formaldehyde, Home Health Complaints, Insulation, Paints, Cleaners and Solvents, Particulates, Pesticides, Radon, Termiticides and Chlordane, and Wood Preservatives

Colorado Department of Health
4210 E 10th Ave
Denver CO 80220
303-331-8500

CONNECTICUT

Asbestos, Biologicals, Home Health Complaints, Insulation, Lead (in paint), Odors, Particulates, Pesticides, Radon, Termiticides and Chlordane, Wood Preservatives

Connecticut Department of Health Services
150 Washington St
Hartford CT 06106
203-556-3186

Formaldehyde, Paints, Solvents, Cleaners

Lois Bryant
Connecticut Department of Consumer Protection
165 Capitol Ave
Hartford CT 06106
203-556-2274

DELAWARE

Asbestos

Robert Foster
Occupational Safety and Health
Delaware Department of Administrative Services
P.O. Box 1401
Dover DE 19903
302-739-5261

Biologicals, Formaldehyde, Insulation, Paints, Solvents and Cleaners, Radon

Bureau of Environmental Health
Division of Public Health
Delaware Department of Health and Social Services
Federal and Water
P.O. Box 637, Jesse Cooper Building
Dover DE 19901
302-739-3028

Odors

Enforcement Section
Department of Natural Resources and
   Environmental Control
89 Kings Highway
Dover DE 19901
302-739-4764

Pesticides, Termiticides, Chlordane, Wood Preservatives
Grier Stayton
Delaware Department of Agriculture
2320 S Du Pont Highway
Dover DE 19901
302-739-4811

DISTRICT OF COLUMBIA

Asbestos, Biologicals, Formaldehyde, Lead (in paint), Odors, Paints, Solvents and Cleaners, Particulates, Wood Preservatives
Air Quality Control and Maintenance Branch
Environmental Control Division
District of Columbia Department of Consumer and
    Regulatory Affairs
2100 Martin Luther King Blvd SE
Washington DC 20020
202-404-1180

Home Health Complaints
Lorenzo White
District of Columbia Department of Employment Services
Occupational Safety and Health
950 Upshur St
Washington DC 20011
202-576-6339

Insulation
Jai Gupta
District of Columbia Energy Office
613 G Street NW Suite 500
Washington DC 20001
202-727-4700

Radon
Norma Stewart
Service Facilities Regulation Administration
District of Columbia Department of Consumer and
    Regulatory Affairs
614 H Street NW
Washington DC 20001
202-727-7218

FLORIDA

Asbestos, Biologicals, Odors, Particulates

Florida Department of Environmental Regulation
2600 Blair Stone Rd
Tallahassee FL 32399
904-488-1344

Formaldehyde, Home Health Complaints, Insulation, Lead (in paint), Paint, Solvents and Cleaners, Pesticides, Radon, Termiticides and Chlordane, Wood Preservatives

Florida Department of Health and
    Rehabilitative Services
1317 Winewood Blvd
Tallahassee FL 32399
904-488-3385

GEORGIA

Asbestos, Biologicals, Formaldehyde, Insulation, Odors, Particulates

Jim Dinnon
Division of Public Health
Georgia Department of Human Resources
878 Peachtree St NE Room 200
Atlanta GA 30309
404-894-6644

Pesticides, Termiticides, Chlordane, Wood Preservatives

Georgia Department of Agriculture
19 Martin Luther King Dr SW
Atlanta GA 30334
404-656-4958

Radon

Tom Hill
Environmental Protection Division
Georgia Department of Natural Resources
Floyd Towers East Suite 1166
205 Butler St SE
Atlanta GA 30334
404-894-5795

GUAM

Asbestos, Biological Complaint Investigations, Odors
Division of Environmental Health
Guam Department of Public Health and
  Social Services
P.O. Box 2816
Agana GU 96910
671-734-7220/210

Combustion Devices and Gases, Formaldehyde, Insulation, Paints, Cleaners and Solvents, Particulates, Pesticides, Radon, Termiticides, Chlordane, Wood Preservatives
Guam Environmental Protection Agency
Government of Guam
D-107 Harmon Plaza
130 Rojas St
Harmon GU 96911
671-734-7305

HAWAII

Asbestos, Biologicals, Formaldehyde, Home Health Complaints, Odors, Particulates, Radon
Hawaii Department of Health
1250 Punchbowl St
Honolulu HI 96813
808-543-8200

Insulation
Philip Dol
Hawaii Office of Consumer Protection
828 Fort St 600B
Honolulu HI 96813
808-548-4091

Pesticides, Termiticides, Chlordane, Wood Preservatives
Hawaii Department of Agriculture
Division of Plant Industry
1428 S King St
P.O. Box 22159
Honolulu HI 96823
808-548-7124

IDAHO

Asbestos, Formaldehyde, Health Complaints, Pesticides, Radon, Termiticides, Chlordane, Wood Preservatives

Idaho Department of Health and Welfare
Statehouse Mall
Boise ID 83720
208-334-5898

Insulation

Wayne Larsen
Idaho Department of Labor and Industrial Services
Building Division
227 N Sixth St
Statehouse Mall
Boise ID 83720
208-334-3896

ILLINOIS

Asbestos, Biologicals, Combustion Devices and Gases, Formaldehyde, Home Health Complaints, Insulation, Lead (in paint), Odors, Paints, Solvents and Cleaners, Particulates, Pesticides, Radon, Termiticides, Chlordane, Wood Preservatives

Illinois Department of Public Health
525 W Jefferson St
Springfield IL 62761
215-782-5830

INDIANA

Asbestos, Biologicals, Formaldehyde, Home Health Complaints, Insulation, Lead (in paint), Paints, Solvents and Cleaners, Particulates, Radon, Termiticides, Chlordane

Indiana State Board of Health
1330 W Michigan St
P.O. Box 1964
Indianapolis IN 46206-1964
317-633-0100

Combustion Devices and Gases

David L. Bills
Indiana Department of Fire and Building Services
Division of Technical Services and Research
1099 N Meridian St Ste 900
Indianapolis IN 46204
317-232-1402

IOWA

Asbestos, Biologicals, Formaldehyde, Home Health Complaints, Insulation, Odors, Particulates, Radon

Iowa Department of Public Health
Division of Disease Prevention
Lucas State Office Building
Des Moines IA 50319
515-281-7785

Pesticides, Termiticides, Chlordane, Wood Preservatives

Charles Eckerman
Iowa Department of Agriculture and
    Land Stewardship
Pesticide Bureau
Wallace State Office Building
Des Moines IA 50319
515-281-8591

KANSAS

Asbestos, Biologicals, Formaldehyde, Home Health Complaints, Insulation, Odors, Particulates, Radon

Kansas Department of Health and Environment
109 SW Ninth St
Topeka KS 66620
913-296-1543

Pesticides, Termiticides, Chlordane

Kansas Board of Agriculture
Plant Health Division
109 SW Ninth St
Topeka KS 66612
913-296-5192

KENTUCKY

Asbestos, Biologicals, Combustion Devices and Gases, Formaldehyde, Home Health Complaints, Insulation, Odors, Paints, Solvents and Cleaners, Particulates, Pesticides, Termiticides, Chlordane, Wood Preservatives

Kentucky Department for Environmental Protection
Division for Air Quality
316 St. Clair Mall
Frankfort KY 40601
502-564-3382

Lead (in paint), Radon

Division of Community Safety
Department for Health Services
Kentucky Cabinet for Human Resources
275 E Main St
Frankfort KY 40621-0001
502-564-3700

LOUISIANA

Asbestos, Biologicals, Formaldehyde, Home Health Complaints, Insulation, Paints, Solvents and Cleaners, Particulates, Pesticides, Radon, Termiticides, Chlordane, Wood Preservatives

Louisiana Department of Health and Hospitals
Office of Public Health Services
Environmental Epidemiology
P.O. Box 60630
New Orleans LA 70160
504-568-2514

Odors

Gus von Bodungen
Department of Environmental Quality
Air Quality Division
P.O. Box 44066
Baton Rouge LA 70804
504-342-1201

MAINE

Asbestos, Biologicals, Combustion Devices and Gases, Odors, Paints, Solvents and Cleaners, Particulates, Radon

Henry E. Warren
Maine Department of Administration
Statehouse Station 77
Augusta ME 04333
207-289-4509

Formaldehyde, Home Health Complaints, Lead (in paint), Pesticides, Termiticides, Chlordane, Wood Preservatives

Maine Department of Human Services
Bureau of Health
Division of Health Engineering
Indoor Air Program
Statehouse Station 10
Augusta ME 04333
207-289-5689

MARYLAND

Asbestos, Biologicals, Combustion Devices and Gases, Formaldehyde, Home Health Complaints, Insulation, Lead (in paint), Odors, Paints, Solvents and Cleaners, Particulates, Pesticides, Radon, Termiticides, Chlordane, Wood Preservatives

Maryland Department of the Environment
2500 Broening Highway
Baltimore MD 21224
301-631-3834 or 301-631-3300

MASSACHUSETTS

Asbestos, Biologicals, Formaldehyde, Home Health Complaints, Insulation, Odors, Particulates, Pesticides, Radon, Termiticides, Wood Preservatives

Massachusetts Department of Public Health
Division of Community Sanitation
150 Tremont St
Boston MA 02111
617-727-2660

Combustion Devices and Gases, Paints, Solvents and Cleaners

Barbara Kwetz
Massachusetts Department of
  Environmental Protection
Division of Air Quality Control
1 Winter St
Boston MA 02108
617-292-5593

MICHIGAN

*Asbestos, Biologicals, Combustion Devices and Gases,
Formaldehyde, Home Health Complaints, Lead (in paint),
Odors, Paints, Solvents and Cleaners, Particulates, Pesticides,
Radon, Termiticides, Chlordane, Wood Preservatives*

Michigan Department of Public Health
3423 N Lansing St
P.O. Box 30195
Lansing MI 48909
517-335-9218 or 1-800-648-6942 for health complaints

Insulation

Michigan Department of Labor
Bureau of Construction Codes
State Secondary Complex
7150 Harris Dr
P.O. Box 30015
Lansing MI 48909
517-322-1801

MINNESOTA

*Asbestos, Biologicals, Combustion Devices and Gases,
Formaldehyde, Insulation, Home Health Complaints, Lead (in
paint), Odors, Paints, Solvents and Cleaners, Particulates, Radon*

Minnesota Department of Health
P.O. Box 59040
925 SE Delaware St
Minneapolis MN 55459-0040
612-627-5010

Pesticides, Termiticides, Chlordane, Wood Preservatives

Minnesota Department of Agriculture
Division of Agronomy Services
90 W Plato Blvd
St. Paul MN 55107
612-296-8547

MISSISSIPPI

Asbestos

Wayne B. Anderson
Mississippi Department of Natural Resources
Bureau of Pollution Control
Air Quality Branch
Jackson MS 39209
601-961-5171

Biologicals, Formaldehyde, Odors, Paints, Solvents and Cleaners, Radon

Mississippi Department of Health
P.O. Box 1700
Jackson MS 39215-1700
601-960-7725

Pesticides, Termiticides, Chlordane, Wood Preservatives

Mississippi Department of Agriculture and Commerce
Division of Plant Industry
P.O. Box 5207
Mississippi State MS 39762
601-325-3390

MISSOURI

Asbestos, Biologicals, Formaldehyde, Home Health Complaints, Insulation, Lead (in paints), Odors, Paints, Solvents and Cleaners, Particulates, Pesticides, Radon, Termiticides, Chlordane, Wood Preservatives

Missouri Department of Health
1730 E Elm St
P.O. Box 570
Jefferson City MO 65102-0570
314-751-6080

Combustion Devices and Gases

Jerzy Wilus
Division of Energy
Department of Natural Resources
P.O. Box 176
Jefferson City MO 65102
314-751-4000

MONTANA

Asbestos, Biologicals, Combustion Devices and Gases, Home Health Complaints, Formaldehyde, Insulation, Odors, Paints, Solvents and Cleaners, Particulates, Pesticides, Radon, Termiticides, Chlordane, Wood Preservatives

Montana Department of Health and
  Environmental Sciences
Cogswell Building
Helena MT 59620
406-444-3986

NEBRASKA

Asbestos, Biologicals, Combustion Devices and Gases, Formaldehyde, Insulation, Odors, Paints, Solvents and Cleaners, Particulates, Pesticides, Radon, Termiticides, Chlordane, Wood Preservatives

Nebraska Department of Health
Bureau of Environmental Health
301 Centennial Mall S
Lincoln NE 68509
402-471-2541

NEVADA

Asbestos, Biologicals, Paints, Cleaners and Solvents, Particulates

Nevada Department of Industrial Relations
Occupational Safety and Health Division
1390 S Curry St
Carson City NV 89710
702-885-3270

Formaldehyde, Radon

Nevada Department of Human Resources
Division of Health
505 E King St
Carson City NV 89710
702-687-4740 or 702-687-5397

Pesticides, Termiticides, Wood Preservatives

Nevada Department of Agriculture
Division of Plant Industry
350 Capitol Hill Ave
Reno NV 89510
702-789-0180

NEW HAMPSHIRE

Asbestos, Biologicals, Combustion Devices and Gases, Formaldehyde, Home Health Complaints, Insulation, Lead (in paint), Odors, Paints, Solvents and Cleaners, Particulates, Radon

New Hampshire Department of Health and
    Human Services
6 Hazen Dr
Concord NH 03301-6527
603-271-4587 or 603-271-4588

Pesticides, Termiticides, Chlordane, Wood Preservatives

New Hampshire Department of Agriculture
Division of Pesticide Control
Caller Box 2042
Concord NH 03301
603-271-3550 or
Health and Human Services
603-271-4664

NEW JERSEY

Asbestos, Biologicals, Combustion Devices and Gases, Formaldehyde, Insulation, Home Health Complaints, Odors, Lead (in paints), Paints, Solvents and Cleaners, Particulates, Pesticides, Radon, Termiticides, Chlordane, Wood Preservatives

New Jersey Department of Health
Department of Occupational and
  Environmental Health
CN 360
Trenton NJ 08625
609-292-5617

NEW MEXICO

Asbestos, Paints, Solvents and Cleaners

Selby Lucero
New Mexico General Services Department
Property Control Division
Joseph Moore Building Rm 2022
1100 St. Francis Dr
Santa Fe NM 87501
505-827-2141

Insulation

Harold J. Trujillo
New Mexico Energy, Mineral and
  Natural Resources Department
Energy Conservation and Management Division
Engineering and Technical Services Bureau
525 Marquez Pl
Santa Fe NM 87501
505-827-5908

Pesticides, Termiticides and Chlordane, Wood Preservatives

Barry E. Peterson
New Mexico Agriculture Department
Agricultural and Environmental Division
P.O. Box 30005 Dept 3150
New Mexico State University
Las Cruces NM 88003-0005
505-646-3208

Radon

William N. Floyd
Environmental Department
Radiation Licensing and Registration Section
P.O. Box 968
Santa Fe NM 87504-0968
505-827-2956

NEW YORK

Asbestos, Biologicals, Formaldehyde, Home Health Complaints, Odors, Paints, Solvents and Cleaners, Particulates, Radon

New York State Department of Health
2 University Place Rm 375
Albany NY 12203-3313
518-458-6461 or
1-800-468-1158 (in New York state)

Pesticides, Termiticides, Chlordane, Wood Preservatives

Marilyn M. DuBois
New York State Department of
  Environmental Conservation
Bureau of Pesticide Management
50 Wolf Rd Rm 404
Albany NY 12223
518-457-7482

NORTH CAROLINA

Asbestos, Biologicals, Combustion Devices and Gases, Formaldehyde, Home Health Complaints, Insulation, Lead (in paint), Odors, Paints, Cleaners and Solvents, Particulates, Pesticides, Radon, Termiticides, Chlordane, Wood Preservatives

North Carolina Department of Environment,
  Health, and Natural Resources
P.O. Box 2091
Raleigh NC 27602
919-733-3680 or 919-733-3410

NORTH DAKOTA

Asbestos, Biologicals, Combustion Devices and Gases, Formaldehyde, Home Health Complaints, Insulation, Odors, Radon

North Dakota Department of Health and
  Consolidated Laboratories
1200 Missouri Ave
P.O. Box 5520
Bismarck ND 58505-5520
701-224-2374 or 701-221-5188

Pesticides, Termiticides, Chlordane, Wood Preservatives

Doug Tollefson
North Dakota Department of Agriculture
Plant Industries Division
State Capitol 6th Floor
Bismarck ND 58505
701-221-5188

OHIO

Asbestos, Biologicals, Formaldehyde, Insulation, Lead (in paint), Odors, Particulates, Pesticides, Radon, Termiticides, Chlordane, Wood Preservatives

Ohio Department of Health
246 N High St
Columbus OH 43266-0588
614-466-1450

OKLAHOMA

Asbestos, Biologicals, Combustion Devices and Gases, Formaldehyde, Home Health Complaints, Insulation, Lead (in paint), Odors, Paints, Solvents and Cleaners, Particulates, Radon

Oklahoma State Department of Health
Consumer Protection Service
1000 NE 10th St
P.O. Box 53551
Oklahoma City OK 73152
405-271-5221

Pesticides, Termiticides, Chlordane, Wood Preservatives
Bob Chada
Oklahoma State Department of Agriculture
Plant Industry Division
Pest Management Section
2800 N Lincoln Blvd
Oklahoma City OK 73105-4298
405-521-3864 or 3871

OREGON

Asbestos, Biologicals, Formaldehyde, Home Health Complaints, Insulation, Lead (in paint), Odors, Particulates, Pesticides, Radon, Termiticides, Wood Preservatives
Oregon Health Division
Oregon Department of Human Resources
1400 SW Fifth Ave
Portland OR 97201
503-229-2572 or 5022

Combustion Devices and Gases
Department of Environmental Quality
811 SW Sixth Ave
Portland OR 97204
503-229-6459

Paints, Solvents and Cleaners
Oregon Occupational Safety and Health Division
Department of Insurance and Finance
Resource Center
Labor and Industries Building
Salem OR 97310
503-378-3272

PENNSYLVANIA

Asbestos, Biologicals, Formaldehyde, Home Health Complaints
Pennsylvania Department of Health
Division of Environmental Health
P.O. Box 90
Harrisburg PA 17108
717-787-1708

Insulation, Odors, Particulates, Radon, Termiticides, Chlordane

Pennsylvania Department of Environmental Resources
Bureau of Air Quality Control
101 S Second St Executive House
P.O. Box 2357
Harrisburg PA 17105-2357
717-787-1663

PUERTO RICO

Asbestos, Biologicals, Combustion Devices and Gases, Odors, Paints, Solvents and Cleaners, Particulates

Puerto Rico Environmental Quality Board
204 Ramaiada St
P.O. Box 11488
Santurce PR 00910
809-725-8898

Radon

David Saidana
Radiological Health Division
Puerto Rico Department of Health
SAMPSF Call Box 70184
San Juan PR 00936
809-767-3561

RHODE ISLAND

Asbestos, Biologicals, Formaldehyde, Home Health Complaints, Insulation, Lead (in paint), Odors, Paints, Solvents and Cleaners, Particulates, Pesticides, Radon, Termiticides, Chlordane

Rhode Island Department of Health
206 Cannon Building
3 Capitol Hill
Providence RI 02908-5097
401-277-2438 or 401-277-3601

SOUTH CAROLINA

Asbestos, Biologicals, Combustion Devices and Gases, Formaldehyde, Insulation, Lead (in paint), Odors, Particulates, Radon

South Carolina Department of Health and
   Environmental Control
2600 Bull St
Columbia SC 29201
803-734-4730

Home Health Complaints, Paints, Solvents and Cleaners

Bill Lybrand
Department of Labor
Occupational Safety and Health Division
3600 Forest Dr
P.O. Box 11329
Columbia SC 29211-1329
803-734-9644

Pesticides, Termiticides, Chlordane, Wood Preservatives

Von H. McCaskill
South Carolina Department of Fertilizer and
   Pesticide Control
256 P&AS Building Clemson University
Clemson SC 29634-0394
803-656-3171

SOUTH DAKOTA

Asbestos, Biologicals, Combustion Devices and Gases, Formaldehyde, Home Health Complaints, Insulation, Lead (in paint), Odors, Paints, Solvents and Cleaners, Particulates, Pesticides, Radon, Termiticides

South Dakota Department of Health
Division of Public Health
Joe Foss Building
523 E Capitol Ave
Pierre SD 57501
605-773-3364

Wood Preservatives

Brad Berven
South Dakota Department of Agriculture
Division of Regulatory Services
Anderson Building
445 E Capitol Ave
Pierre SD 57501
605-773-3724

TENNESSEE

Asbestos, Biologicals, Combustion Devices and Gases, Formaldehyde, Insulation, Odors, Paints, Solvents and Cleaners, Particulates, Radon

Tennessee Department of Health & Environment
Division of Air Pollution Control
Customs House
701 Broadway
Nashville TN 37247-3530
615-741-3931

Home Health and Lead in Paint Complaints

Dr. Sarah Sell
Tennessee Department of Health
Environmental Epidemiology Program
C1-130 Cordell Hull Building
Nashville TN 37247-4912
615-741-5683

Pesticides, Termiticides, Chlordane, Wood Preservatives

Tennessee Department of Agriculture
Plant Industries Division
P.O. Box 40627 Melrose Station
Nashville TN 37204
615-360-0130

TEXAS

Asbestos, Biologicals, Combustion Devices and Gases, Formaldehyde, Home Health Complaints, Lead (in paint), Odors, Paints, Solvents and Cleaners, Particulates, Pesticides, Radon, Termiticides, Chlordane, Wood Preservatives

Texas Department of Health
1100 W 49th St
Austin TX 78704
512-458-7700 or 512-835-7000 (radon)

Insulation

Jimmy G. Martin
Texas Department of Licensing and Regulation
Manufactured Housing Division
P.O. Box 12157
Austin TX 78711
512-436-7357

UTAH

Asbestos, Biologicals, Home Health Complaints, Lead (in paint), Particulates

Utah Department of Health
288 N 1460 W
Salt Lake City UT 84116
801-538-6108

Combustion Devices and Gases, Formaldehyde, Insulation, Radon

Utah Energy Office
355 W North Temple Ste 450
Third Triad Center
Salt Lake City UT 84180-1204
801-538-5428

Pesticides, Termiticides, Chlordane, Wood Preservatives

Van Burgess
Department of Agriculture
Division of Plant Industries
350 N Redwood Rd
Salt Lake City UT 84116
801-533-4107

VERMONT

Asbestos, Biologicals, Formaldehyde, Home Health Complaints, Insulation, Lead (in paint), Odors, Particulates, Paints, Solvents and Cleaners, Radon

Vermont Department of Health
60 Main St
P.O. Box 70
Burlington VT 05402
802-863-7720

Pesticides, Termiticides, Chlordane, Wood Preservatives

Vermont Department of Agriculture
116 State St
State Office Building
Montpelier VT 05602
802-828-2431

VIRGINIA

Asbestos, Biologicals, Combustion Devices and Gases, Formaldehyde, Home Health Complaints, Insulation, Lead (in paint), Odors, Paints, Solvents and Cleaners, Particulates, Pesticides, Radon, Termiticides, Chlordane, Wood Preservatives

Virginia Department of Health
Box 2448
1500 E Main St
Richmond VA 23218
804-786-1763 or 804-786-6029 (biologicals)

WASHINGTON

Asbestos, Biologicals, Formaldehyde, Home Health Complaints, Insulation, Odors, Paints, Solvents and Cleaners, Particulates, Pesticides, Radon, Termiticides, Chlordane, Wood Preservatives

Washington Department of Health
Mall Stop LD-11
Olympia WA 98504
206-586-6179

WEST VIRGINIA

Asbestos, Home Health Complaints, Insulation, Odors, Pesticides, Radon, Termiticides, Chlordane, Wood Preservatives

West Virginia Bureau of Public Health
Office of Environmental Health Services
Industrial Hygiene Division
151 11th Ave
South Charleston WV 25303
304-348-0696

Biologicals, Combustion Devices and Gases, Formaldehyde, Paints, Solvents and Cleaners, Particulates

West Virginia Department of Labor
Safety and Boiler Division
Capitol Complex
Charleston WV 25305
304-348-7890

WISCONSIN

Asbestos, Biologicals, Combustion Devices and Gases, Formaldehyde, Home Health Complaints, Insulation, Lead (in paint), Odors, Paints, Solvents and Cleaners, Particulates, Pesticides, Radon, Termiticides, Chlordane, Wood Preservatives

Wisconsin Department of Health and Social Services
1414 E Washington Ave
Madison WI 53703
608-266-2895 or 608-266-9337 (asbestos)

WYOMING

Formaldehyde, Home Health Complaints, Insulation, Lead (in paint), Radon

Wyoming Department of Health
Hathaway Building
Cheyenne WY 82002

Pesticides, Termiticides, Chlordane, Wood Preservatives

Wyoming Department of Agriculture
Division of Standards and Consumer Services
2219 Carey Ave
Cheyenne WY 82002-0100
307-777-7321

Directory B
U.S. Environmental Protection Agency Regional Office Indoor Air, Radon, and Asbestos Contacts

Address written inquiries to the Indoor Air Contact, Radon Contact, or Asbestos Contact in the EPA Regional offices at the following addresses:

Region

States in Region

Region 1
EPA
JFK Federal Building
Boston MA 02203
617-565-3232 (Indoor Air)
617-565-4502 (Radon)
617-565-3744 (Asbestos)

Connecticut
Maine
Massachusetts
New Hampshire
Rhode Island
Vermont

Region 2
EPA
26 Federal Plaza
New York NY 10278
212-264-2622 (Indoor Air)
212-264-0546 (Radon)
212-264-6770 (Asbestos)

New Jersey
New York
Puerto Rico
Virgin Islands

Region 3
EPA
841 Chestnut Building
Philadelphia PA 19107
215-597-8322 (Indoor Air)
215-597-4084 (Radon)
215-597-3160 (Asbestos)

Delaware
District of Columbia
Maryland
Pennsylvania
Virginia
West Virginia

Region	**States in Region**

Region 4
EPA
345 Courtland St NE
Fourth Floor
Atlanta GA 30365
404-347-2964 (Indoor Air)
404-347-3907 (Radon)
404-347-5014 (Asbestos)

Alabama
Florida
Georgia
Kentucky
Mississippi
North Carolina
South Carolina
Tennessee

Region 5
EPA
230 S Dearborn St
Chicago IL 60604
312-886-6043 (Indoor Air)
312-886-6042 (Radon)
312-353-4425 (Asbestos)

Illinois
Indiana
Michigan
Minnesota
Ohio
Wisconsin

Region 6
EPA
1445 Rose Ave
Dallas TX 75202-2733
214-655-7229 (Indoor Air)
214-655-7223 (Radon)
214-655-7244 (Asbestos)

Arkansas
Louisiana
Oklahoma
New Mexico
Texas

Region 7
EPA
726 Minnesota Ave
Kansas City KS 66101
913-551-7020 (Indoor Air)
913-551-7020 (Radon)
913-551-7020 (Asbestos)

Iowa
Kansas
Missouri
Nebraska

Region 8
EPA
999 18th St Ste 500
Denver CO 80202-2405
303-293-1887 (Indoor Air)
303-293-1713 (Radon)
303-293-1442 (Asbestos)

Colorado
Montana
North Dakota
South Dakota
Utah
Wyoming

Region	**States in Region**
Region 9 EPA 75 Hawthorne St San Francisco CA 94105 415-744-1087 (Indoor Air) 415-744-1085 (Radon) 415-744-1087 (Asbestos)	Arizona California Hawaii Nevada American Samoa Guam Trust Territories of the Pacific
Region 10 EPA 1200 Sixth Ave Seattle WA 98101 206-553-2589 (Indoor Air) 206-553-7660 (Radon) 206-553-4762 (Asbestos)	Alaska Idaho Oregon Washington

Directory C
National Hotlines and Clearing Houses

U.S. Environmental Protection Agency

EPA Radon Hotline (toll-free): 800-SOS-RADO(N), which is 800-767-7236

EPA Radon Public Information: 202-475-9605

EPA Public Information Center: 202-382-2080

National Pesticides Telecommunications Network Hotline (toll-free): 800-858-PEST or 800-858-7378
800-743-3091 in Texas

TSCA Assistance (Toxic Substance and Control Act) Information Service: 202-554-1404

Safe Drinking Water Hotline (toll-free) 800-426-4791

U.S. Consumer Product Safety Commission

Product Safety Hotline (toll-free): 800-638-CPSC or 800-638-2772

U.S. Department of Health and Human Services

NIOSH Public Information (toll-free): 800-35-NIOSH or 800-356-4674

Indoor Air Quality Assurance: 513-841-4382

Center for Environmental Research Information

Central Point of distribution for EPA research results and reports. 513-569-7391 Cincinnati, Ohio

Asbestos Ombudsman

Responds to questions and concerns about asbestos in schools issues. Operates Monday through Friday, 8:00 A.M.–4:30 P.M.
800-368-5888
557-1938 in the Washington, D.C. area

Emergency Planning and Community Right-to-Know Information Hotline

Provides communities and individuals with help in preparing for accidental releases of toxic chemicals. This hotline, which compliments the RCRA/Superfund Hotline, is maintained as an in-

formation resource rather than an emergency number. Operates Monday through Friday from 8:30 A.M. to 7:30 P.M. Eastern Time.
800-535-0202
479-2449 in the Washington, D.C. area

Hazardous Waste Ombudsman

Assists citizens and the regulated community that have had problems voicing a complaint or getting a problem resolved about hazardous waste issues. There is a Hazardous Waste Ombudsman at EPA Headquarters and one in each of the EPA's 10 Regional Offices.
202-475-9361 Washington, D.C.

Inspector General's Whistle Blower Hotline

This hotline is for reporting EPA-related waste, fraud, abuse, or mismanagement. Operates Monday through Friday from 10:00 A.M. to 3:00 P.M. Eastern Time. At other times, callers may leave a message.
800-424-4000
382-4977 in the Washington, D.C. area

National Pesticides Telecommunications Network Hotline

Provides information on pesticide-related health, toxicity, and minor cleanup to physicians, veterinarians, fire departments, government agencies, and the general public. Also provides impartial information on pesticide products, basic safety practices, health and environmental effects, and cleanup and disposal procedures. The hotline is staffed by pesticide specialists at Texas Tech University's School of Medicine. Operates 24 hours a day, 365 days a year.
800-858-7378
806-743-3091 in Texas

National Poison Control Center Hotline

Operated by Georgetown University Hospital in Washington, D.C., this hotline provides information on accidental ingestion of chemicals, poisons, or drugs.
202-625-3333 Washington, D.C.

National Response Center Hotline

Operated by the U.S. Coast Guard, this hotline is used to report spills of oil and other hazardous materials. The hotline is available 24 hours a day, every day of the year.
800–424–8802
426–2675 in the Washington, D.C. area

National Small Flows Clearinghouse

Provides information on wastewater treatment technologies for small communities.
800–624–8301

Pollution Prevention Information Clearinghouse

Provides information and answers to questions about reducing or eliminating discharges and/or emissions to the environment through source reduction and environmentally sound recycling.
800–424–9346
202–382–3000 in the Washington, D.C. area

Radon Information

For information about radon, you should call the Radon Office in your individual state. In the Washington, D.C. area, the numbers are:
Maryland 800–872–3666
Virginia 800–468–0138
Washington, D.C. 202–727–7728

The Radon Office at EPA Headquarters responds to requests for information on radon issues.
202–475–9605 Washington, D.C.

RCRA/CERCLA (Superfund) Hotline

Responds to questions from the public and regulated community on the Resource Conservation and Recovery Act, and the Comprehensive Environmental Response, Compensation, and Liability Act (Superfund). Responds to requests for RCRA and Superfund documents. Operates Monday through Friday from 8:30 A.M. to 7:30 P.M. Eastern Time.
800–424–9346
202–382–3000 in the Washington, D.C. area

Safe Drinking Water Hotline

Provides information and publications to the public and regulated community concerning EPA's drinking water regulations and programs. Operates Monday through Friday, 8:30 A.M. to 4:30 P.M. Eastern Time.
800-426-4791
382-5533 in the Washington, D.C. area

Small Business Ombudsman Hotline

Assists small businesses in complying with environmental laws and EPA regulations. Operates Monday through Friday, 8:00 A.M. to 4:30 P.M. Eastern Time. There are also Small Business Ombudsmen in each of EPA's 10 Regional Offices.
800-368-5888
557-1938 in the Washington, D.C. area

Toxic Substances Control Act (TSCA) Assistance Information Service

Provides both general and technical information and publications about toxic substances, including asbestos. A variety of other services are also offered to help businesses comply with TSCA laws, including regulatory advice and aid, publications, and audiovisual materials. Operates Monday through Friday from 8:30 A.M. to 5:00 P.M. Eastern Time.
202-554-1404 Washington, D.C.

Directory D
Resource List of Private Sector and Nonprofit Organizations

Here are some home health and safety sources not listed elsewhere which you can write for additional information:

- The American Lung Association (ALA) has produced a 23-minute slide-tape program, "Air Pollution in Your Home," which may be rented. The ALA has also produced several noteworthy free brochures available to the public: "Air Pollution in Your Home?" "Home Indoor Air Quality Checklist" "Facts About Radon: The Health Risk Indoors" and "Formaldehyde Fact Sheet." Write: Ron White, ALA, 1740 Broadway, New York NY 10019; or phone 212-315-8700.

- Environmental Health Watch (EHW) is a nonprofit organization that educates and assists families concerned about the adverse effects of asbestos, formaldehyde, lead, pesticides, and other toxic substances and products in the home. Write: EHW, 4115 Bridge Ave, Cleveland OH 44113.

- Environmentals Hazards Management Institute (EHMI) has a useful "Household Hazardous Waste Wheel," a color door or cupboard reference that lists the potential hazards of chemical products and offers nontoxic alternatives. Cost is $3.75 to: EHMI, P.O. Box 932, Durham NH 03824; or call 603-868-1496.

- Housing Resource Center (HRC) is a nonprofit organization providing consumers and professionals with practical home maintenance, home improvement, and repair information through its telephone hotline and its publications, including *House-Mending Resources,* a quarterly journal, and *Your Home,* a monthly newsletter. HRC also cosponsors the annual Blueprint for a Healthy House Conference. Contact: HRC, 1820 W. 48th St, Cleveland OH 44102; or call 216-281-4663.

Other private sector organizations that provide information to the public on home health and safety:

- American Institute of Architects, 1350 New York Ave NW, Washington DC 20006

- American Gas Association, 1515 Wilson Blvd, Arlington VA 22209
- American Lung Association, 1740 Broadway, New York NY 10019
- Consumer Federation of America, 1424 16th St NW Ste 604, Washington DC 20036
- Edison Electric Institute, 1111 19th St NW, Washington DC 20036
- National Association of Home Builders, Technology and Codes Department, 15th and M Streets NW, Washington DC 20005
- World Health Organization, Publications Center, 49 Sheridan Ave, Albany NY 12210

INDEX